Pani
FILARIASIS

Pani's FILARIASIS

THIRD EDITION

Sankarsan Pani MBBS (Hons) MS (Surgery)
Ex-Director
Shree Jagannath Dental College
Shree Jagannath Homeopathic Medical College
Ramanandacharya Medical College and Hospital
and Shree Jagannath Hospital
Puri, Odisha, India

Presently
Associate Professor
Mahatma Gandhi Mission's Medical College
Kamothe, Navi Mumbai, Maharashtra, India

Foreword
Mahendrakar

JAYPEE BROTHERS MEDICAL PUBLISHERS (P) LTD

New Delhi • London • Philadelphia • Panama

Jaypee Brothers Medical Publishers (P) Ltd

Headquarters

Jaypee Brothers Medical Publishers (P) Ltd
4838/24, Ansari Road, Daryaganj
New Delhi 110 002, India
Phone: +91-11-43574357
Fax: +91-11-43574314
Email: jaypee@jaypeebrothers.com

Overseas Offices

J.P. Medical Ltd
83 Victoria Street, London
SW1H 0HW (UK)
Phone: +44-2031708910
Fax: +02-03-0086180
Email: info@jpmedpub.com

Jaypee Brothers Medical Publishers Ltd
The Bourse
111 South Independence Mall East
Suite 835, Philadelphia, PA 19106, USA
Phone: + 267-519-9789
Email: joe.rusko@jaypeebrothers.com

Jaypee Brothers Medical Publishers (P) Ltd
Shorakhute, Kathmandu
Nepal
Phone: +00977-9841528578
Email: jaypee.nepal@gmail.com

Jaypee-Highlights Medical Publishers Inc.
City of Knowledge, Bld. 237, Clayton
Panama City, Panama
Phone: +507-301-0496
Fax: +507-301-0499
Email: cservice@jphmedical.com

Jaypee Brothers Medical Publishers (P) Ltd
17/1-B Babar Road, Block-B, Shaymali
Mohammadpur, Dhaka-1207
Bangladesh
Mobile: +08801912003485
Email: jaypeedhaka@gmail.com

Website: www.jaypeebrothers.com
Website: www.jaypeedigital.com

Inquiries for bulk sales may be solicited at: jaypee@jaypeebrothers.com

Pani's Filariasis

First Edition: 1980
Second Edition: 2001
Third Edition: **2013**

ISBN 978-93-5090-477-0

Printed at Rajkamal Electric Press, Plot No. 2, Phase-IV, Kundli, Haryana.

Dedicated to

My Parents

MAHATMA GANDHI MISSION'S
MEDICAL COLLEGE, & HOSPITAL
Sector-18, Kamothe, Navi Mumbai- 410209
Tel: 27422459, 27421723, Fax, 91- 22-7420320

Foreword

I, Dr Mahendrakar know Dr S Pani for the last 7 years.

I have gone through this book and as per my knowledge goes, I know this is the only book in medical science in the topic of filariasis. This book will be very beneficial for the students of medical science and treating physicians.

He has done a lot of work in this field with utmost sincerity and dedication.

I wish him all success in life.

Mahendrakar MS (Gen Surg) MS (Ant)
Professor Emeritus
Department of Anatomy
Mahatma Gandhi Mission Institute of Health Sciences
Kamothe, Navi Mumbai, Maharashtra, India

Preface to the Third Edition

After a gap of 12 years it is decided to have third edition of Pani's Filariasis as there is lot of work has been done in this field. Government of India as well as State Governments are providing lot of assistance to control this disease particularly in costal districts of India.

Nowadays it is found, this disease has equally spreaded in all parts of India. During my short stay in Mahatma Gandhi Mission's (MGM) Medical College, Kamothe, Navi Mumbai, Maharashtra, India, I found lot of patients of filariasis and I have already brought it to the knowledge to the college authority.

I hope this edition will help my professional friends if they take the help of this book.

Sankarsan Pani

Preface to the First Edition

When I was working as a House Surgeon at Maharaja Krishna Chandra Gajapati (MKCG) Medical College, Berhampur, Odisha, India. I was attached to 4th surgical ward of this hospital. Many patients of filariasis were getting admission to this hospital and almost in each case we were referring to our Professor for clarification of our doubts. No definite book was available on this subject at that time. Hence, it was a necessity of publishing a separate book on filariasis. Filariasis is a disease which is mainly seen in states like West Bengal, Odisha, Andhra Pradesh, Tamil Nadu, Kerala, Karnataka, Maharashtra and Gujarat though this is partially distributed all over India. For the sake of medical students of India such a book is a dire necessity which was felt by me during my house-surgeonship. My dream came true while I was practicing at Employees' State Insurance (ESI) Hospital, Choudwar, Odisha, India as a Surgical Specialist.

A filarial clinic was opened at ESI Cottage Hospital, Choudwar during 1978 under my guidance to study the effects of asperzine in the treatment of filariasis. This medicine was compared with diethylcarbamazine in nearly 200 cases. To open the clinic at ESI Hospital, Choudwar, Dr (Major) Gouramohan Mishra, Ex-Director of ESI Scheme of Odisha had taken maximum pains and had requested Labor Department of Government of Odisha as well as ESI Corporation of Government of India to sanction Rs. 2,000/- initially. This request was sympathetically considered and the clinic started functioning from the month of June 1978 and I had to work from 7 pm to 10 pm every Saturday of every week in addition to my usual work. Again Rs. 10,000/- was sanctioned by the same authorities on my request to purchase asperzine. The work could not be completed as I was transferred from ESI Hospital, Choudwar to ESI Hospital, Jaykaypur, Odisha on political pressure.

However, I am highly grateful to Dr (Major) GM Mishra, Ex-Director of ESI Scheme, Odisha; Dr VM Charnalia, Medical Commissioner, ESI Corporation of India and Secretary to Government of Odisha in Labor Department, because of their financial help rendered to me to run the clinic. It will be an injustice if I do not extend my gratefulness and thanks to Sri SC Jain, MSc, FICS, Vice-President (Works) and Sri RN Srinivastava, MA, LLB, General Manager (Mill Administration) of JK Paper Mills, Jaykaypur, because of their benevolent help and guidance from time to time in many forms, without which this book could not have been published.

Lastly, I will be extending my thanks to the Medical College Students and Doctors if they utilize this book for the benefit of humankind. Suggestions, corrections and alterations if any are highly solicited by me for near future.

Sankarsan Pani

Contents

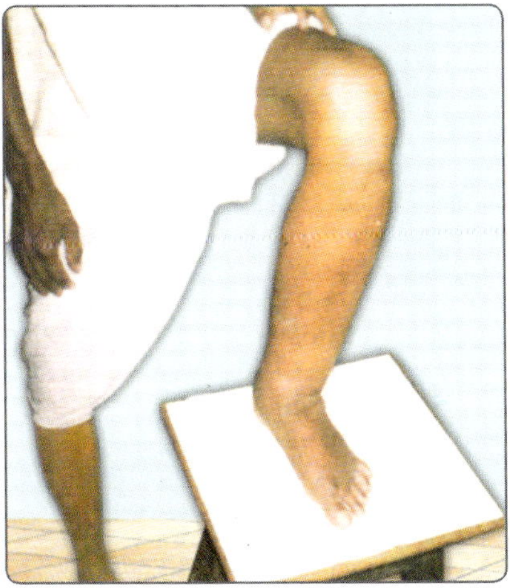

Fig. 3.1: Nonpitting edema

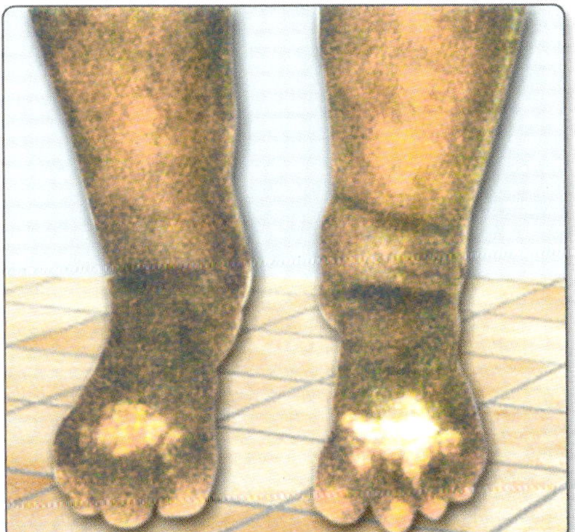

Fig. 3.2: Nonpitting edema

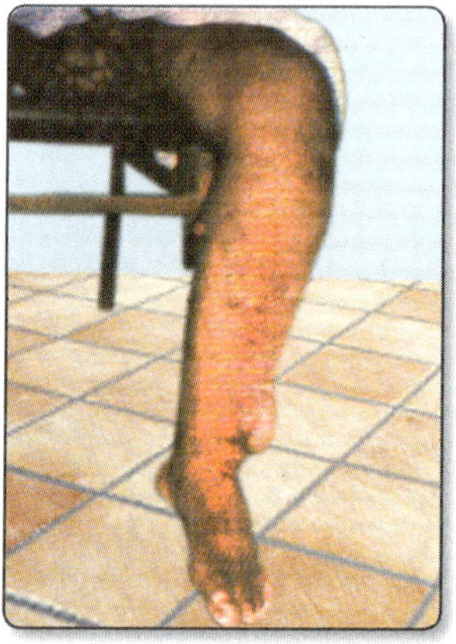

Fig. 6.1: Hydrocele of scrotum

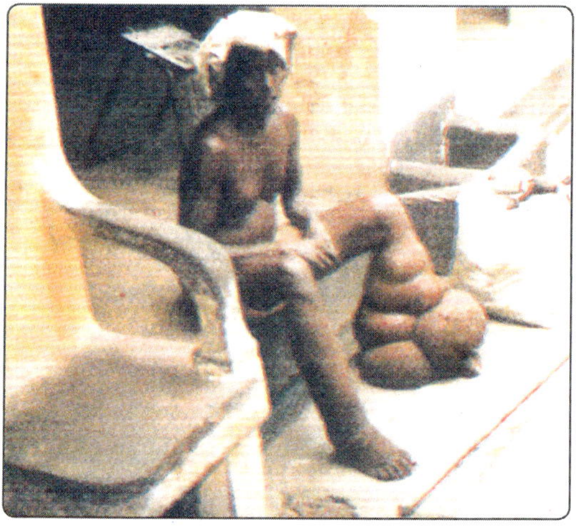

Fig. 6.2: Elephantiasis of limbs
(lymph accumulates in infected limb)

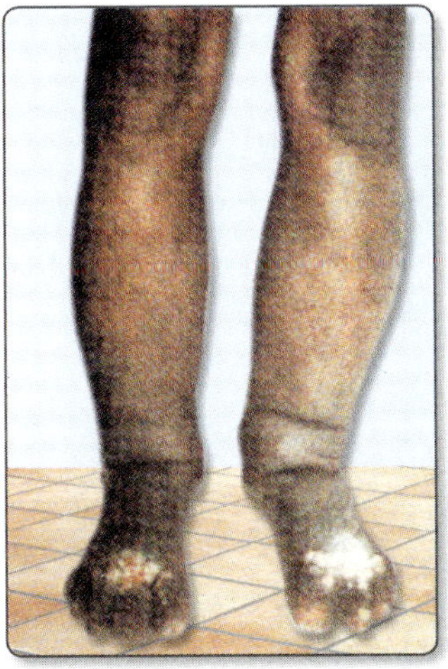

Fig. 6.3: Elephantiasis limb (Fibrotic ulcer)

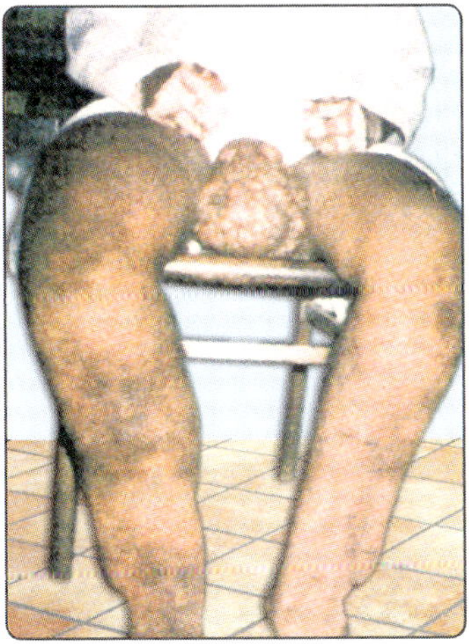

Fig. 6.4: Scrotal abscess

Plate 4

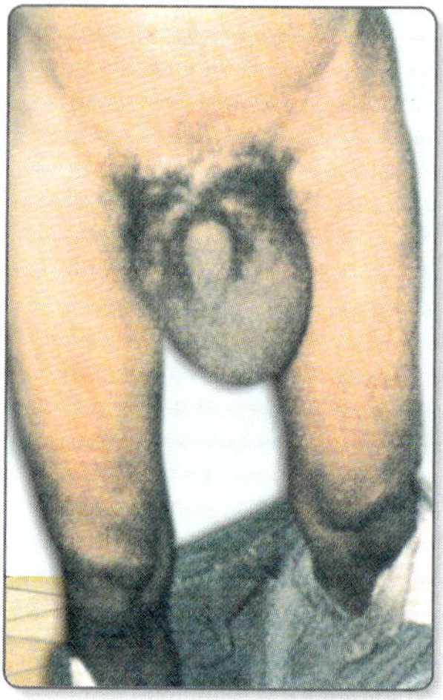

Fig. 7.1: Vaginal hydrocele

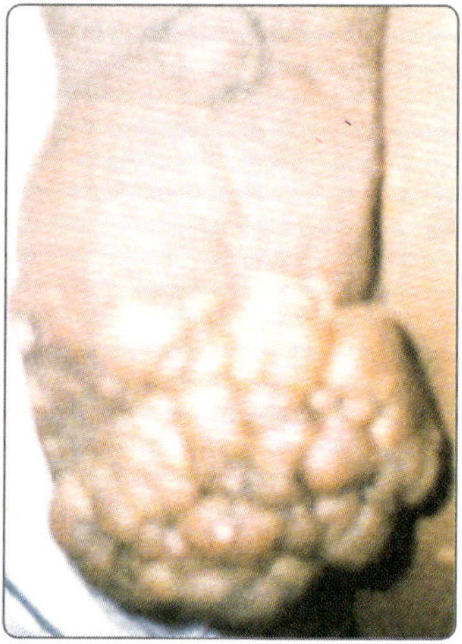

Fig. 7.2: Hydrocele due to filariasis

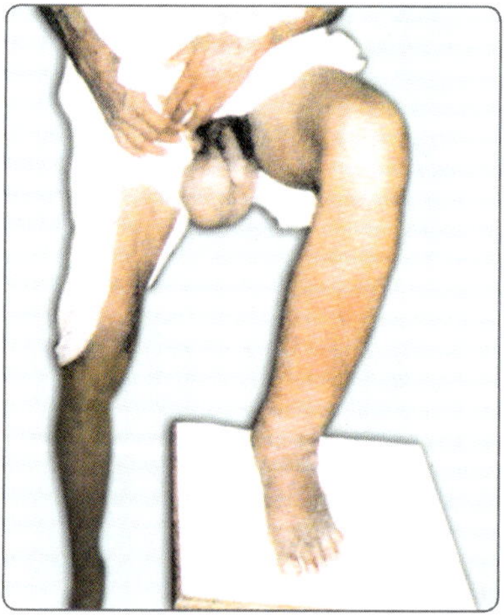

Fig. 7.3: Old hematocele

chapter 1

Anatomy of Lymphatic System

As the filariasis is a primary disease of lymphatic system it is essential to explain the anatomy of lymphatic system before going to filariasis per se. The adult worm of filariasis produces its pathogenesis in lymphatic system only when it enters this system. The microfilaria can enter into skin, blood circulation as well as lymphatic circulation but it manifests the pathogenesis only when it enters the lymphatic circulation. Hence it is necessary to explain the anatomy of lymphatic system keeping the pathogenesis of filariasis in mind. For detailed study of lymphatic system, the reader may refer to a textbook of anatomy. The lymph nodes affected in filariasis in frequency are as follows:

1. Lymph nodes draining lower limb
2. Lymph nodes draining upper limbs
3. Abdominal lymph nodes
4. Thoracic lymph nodes and thoracic duct
5. Lymph nodes of cervical region (very rare).

LYMPHATICS OF LOWER LIMB

The lymph nodes draining the lymph of lower limb are distributed in inguinal region and in popliteal region. By inguinal region it means the lymph nodes are distributed near about inguinal ligament, and that of popliteal region is in popliteal fossa.

Inguinal Lymph Nodes

The inguinal lymph nodes are classified as:

1. Superficial inguinal lymph nodes:
   a. Upper (Transverse) group.
   b. Lower (Longitudinal) group.
2. Deep inguinal lymph nodes.

Superficial Inguinal Lymph Nodes

They are usually present superficial to the deep fascia (Fascia lata) of thigh in inguinal region. This group of lymph nodes are arranged in two sets like upper or transverse group and lower or longitudinal group. The upper group lymph nodes are distributed in parallel with inguinal ligament and they are usually 5 to 6 in number. They are sub-divided in 3 sets like (from lateral to medial) superficial circumflex iliac, superficial epigastric and superficial external pudendal. These sub-groups are named as they are present with corresponding veins in inguinal region. The lower group are 2 to 4 in number and are distributed in parallel with terminal part of long saphenous vein.

Deep Inguinal Lymph Nodes

They are present deep to fascia lata (deep fascia of thigh) and they are usually 1 to 3 in number. The lowest one is present in the lower angle formed at the union of long saphenous vein with femoral vein. The middle one is present in the femoral canal and this lymph node is otherwise named as gland of cloquet. The highest one is present lateral to the femoral ring and may be frequently absent.

The inguinal lymph nodes drain, the lower limb, penis and scrotum (except testis) (external genitalia below hymen in female), gluteal region, anal region, perianal region and adjoining part of abdominal wall below umbilicus.

Popliteal Lymph Nodes

The popliteal lymph nodes are embedded inside the popliteal pad of fat. They are usually 6 to 7 in number. One lymph node is constantly present in the angle formed by the union of short saphenous vein with popliteal vein and another present between posterior surface of knee joint and popliteal artery. Other nodes are present besides the popliteal vessels.

LYMPHATICS OF UPPER LIMB

The lymphatics of upper limb mainly drain into the lymph nodes situated in axilla. The lymphatics are arranged in two sets in upper limb, like superficial and deep. The deep set usually accompanies the neurovascular bundle of upper limb, whereas the superficial set follows the superficial veins of upper limb. However, they are terminated at axillary lymph nodes. The axillary lymph nodes are arranged in 5 groups such as:

Anterior (Pectoral) Group

These are usually 4 to 5 in number and present on the lower boarder of pectoralis minor in relation to lateral thoracic vessels.

Posterior (Subcapular) Group

These are about 6 to 7 in number and situated on the lower boarder of posterior axillary fold in relation to subcapular vessels.

Lateral (Humeral) Group

These are 4 to 6 in number and situated along the course of axillary vein, nearer to the neck of humerus.

Central Group

This group of lymph nodes numbering 4 to 5, embedded in the fat present at the base of axilla. The above sets of lymph nodes drain to this group of lymph nodes. In addition to the above afferent lymphatics, this group also receives afferent lymphatic from breast as well as from back of the body as low as iliac crest.

Apical Group

This group is highest in number (6 to 12) as well as in position. These are present in a triangle, formed by 1st rib medially, axillary vein posteriorly and clavicle anteriorly. The central group of lymph nodes drain to this group of lymph nodes. The efferent lymphatics from these lymph nodes form the subclavian trunk which drains to either at the junction of internal jugular vein with subclavian vein or thoracic duct on left side (or jugular trunk on right side).

In addition to these lymph nodes there are other groups of lymph nodes which are distributed in the course of lymphatics. They are:

a. Supratrochlear lymph nodes—They are 2 to 3 in number and situated on the medial side of humerous above medial epicondyle along the course of basalic vein.
b. Infraclavicular lymph nodes—These lymph nodes are 1 to 2 in number and placed in the infraclavicular fossa along the course of cephalic vein.
c. In addition to the above lymph nodes there may be occasional isolated lymph nodes distributed along with different vessels like ulnar, radial, and brachial. The axillary group of lymph nodes drain the area like upper limb, anterior and posterior surfaces of chest wall including breast, anterior wall of abdomen as below as umbilicus and back of the body as below as iliac crest.

LYMPHATICS OF ABDOMEN AND PELVIS

The lymph node of abdominal cavity and pelvis are arranged in different orders from individual to individual (Flow chart 1.1). The abdomen and pelvis contain a large number of lymph nodes and is second in position. Out of 800 lymph nodes present in the body, the abdomen and pelvis nearly contain 200 of such lymph nodes. All organs of abdomen and pelvis are drained by the lymph nodes of abdomen and pelvis and return to the veins in neck via the thoracic duct. For better appreciation of lymph nodes in the abdomen and pelvis, a classification of lymph nodes is given below. The lymph nodes are primarily described in relation with abdominal aorta and its branches, hence they are as follows:

Preaortic Lymph Nodes

The preaortic lymph nodes are arranged mainly along the branches of coeliac trunk, superior mesenteric and inferior mesenteric arteries. They are classified as per their position of the draining organ. The organs drained by these groups of lymph nodes are: diaphragm, lower part of oesophagus, stomach, duodenum, jejunum, ileum, appendix, colon, rectum, spleen, pancreas, liver, gall bladder and their peritoneal coverings.

Para-aortic Lymph Nodes

These lymph nodes are arranged on both sides of abdominal aorta till to its termination. The organs drained by the main para-aortic lymph nodes are: kidneys, suprarenal gland, testis (ovaries), ureters, partly bladder, and partly uterus. The terminal para-aortic lymph nodes are mainly concerned with drainage of pelvic organs like, bladder, uterus, rectum, vagina, deep structure of perineum as well as pelvic wall.

Retro-aortic Lymph Nodes

Topographically there is no separate group of lymph nodes which are placed behind the aorta. These are mainly included in para-aortic group. These groups of lymph nodes are mainly placed in retro-peritoneal space. The posterior abdominal wall is mainly drained by these groups of lymph nodes. However, all abdominal and pelvic lymph nodes are inter-connected by lymphatic channels, even they also bear interconnecting relations with axillary and inguinal nodes.

LYMPHATICS OF THORAX AND THORACIC DUCT

It has been already explained that the superficial tissues of thoracic wall are drained by the axillary group of lymph nodes but the deep tissues are drained by the following lymph nodes.

Flow chart 1.1: Lymph nodes drained by internal tissues.

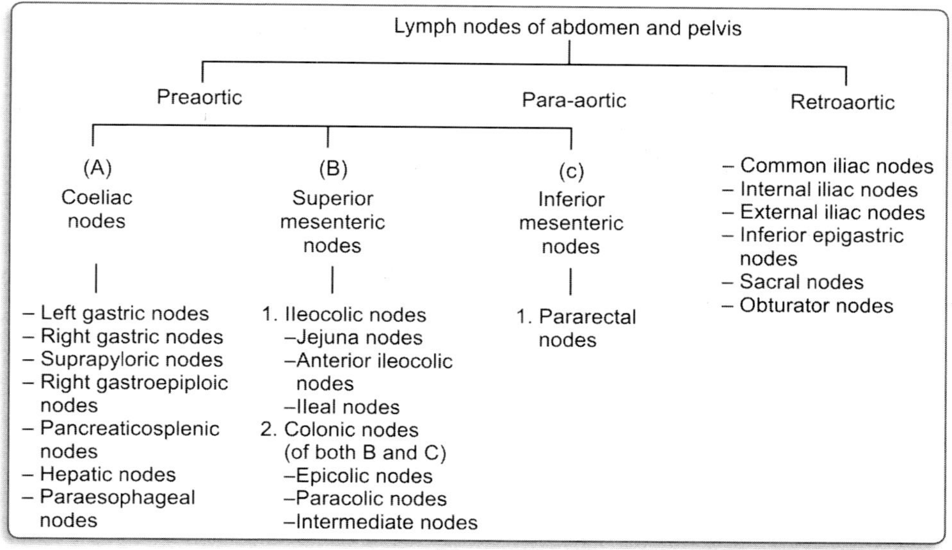

Parasternal Lymph Nodes (Internal Thoracic)

These are 4 to 5 in number and are placed on each side of sternum inside the intercostal space in relation to internal mammary vessels (internal thoracic). The efferent lymphatics from these lymph nodes unite with the lymphatics of the mediastinum to form the jugular trunk (bronchomediastinal trunk) which opens at the junction of right subclavian vein with right internal jugular vein.

Intercostal Lymph Nodes

These lymph nodes are present in each intercostal space in relation to the neck of each ribs. The efferent lymphatics of these nodes drain to the thoracic duct in lower 4 to 5 spaces as-well-as left upper spaces, whereas the jugular trunk receives the efferent lymphatics from the rest of left upper spaces.

Diaphragmatic Lymph Nodes

These lymph nodes are arranged on the circumference of diaphragm in four sets such as anterior, lateral (right and left) and posterior. They all drain into thoracic duct.

The lymphatic drainage of the thoracic contents is performed by the lymph nodes present in the mediastinum. They are as follows:

Superior Mediastinal Lymph Nodes (Brachiocephalic)

These lymph nodes are 20 to 35 in number. They are placed surrounding the brachiocephalic vein in superior mediastinum. They mainly drain to either thoracic duct or jugular trunk.

Anterior Mediastinal (Parasternal) Lymph Nodes

They have been described earlier.

Middle Mediastinal (Tracheobronchial) Lymph Nodes

These lymph nodes are many in number and arranged surrounding trachea as well as bronchi. They are classified as per their position.

Paratracheal (left and right) type: These are present on the side of trachea in tracheoesophageal groove.

Tracheobronchial type (superior and inferior): These lymph nodes are present above and below the principal bronchus. There may be 2 or 3 large nodes placed below the Carina.

Bronchopulmonary type: These lymph nodes are present just in the hilus of each lung.

Pulmonary type: These are present inside the substance of the lung on the course of the bronchus. All of the above lymph nodes drain mainly lungs and heart. On the left side the efferent lymphatics.

Posterior, Mediastinal Lymph Nodes

These are present behind the pericardium in relation to oesophagus and thoracic aorta. It is very much difficult to differentiate between posterior mediastinal and intercostal lymph nodes as these are placed nearer to each other.

THORACIC DUCT

The thoracic duct is the main canal through which major lymph conveys into blood. This duct drains the lymph from below diaphragm, left of chest wall, left side of face and neck, left upper limb as well as left organs of thoracic cavity. It is one of the 18 inches (45 cm) structures. It begins from abdomen and ends in neck. It starts from upper end of cisterna chyli which is placed over 1st and 2nd lumbar vertebrae. Hence, the thoracic duct starts from lower boarder of 12th thoracic vertebra and enters the thoracic cavity through the aortic opening in diaphragm. It ascends through the posterior mediastinum between thoracic aorta on its left and azygous vein on its right. In posterior mediastinum it remains anterior to lower thoracic vertebral column, hemiazygous vein and right intercostal arteries and posterior to oesophagus. At the level of 5th thoracic vertebra it turns to left side and enters the superior mediastinum. Here, it lies behind arch of aorta, left subclavian artery and apex of left lung. In the left side of neck it lies behind left common carotid artery left internal jugular vein and left vagus nerve. Here also it relates anterior to left phrenic nerve, sympathetic trunk and thyrocervical trunk. Then it opens into the junction of left subclavian vein with left internal jugular vein. This corresponds at the level of seventh cervical vertebra. The thoracic duct is segmented by the provision of one way valves in it. Because of its multiple connections with the lymphatics of chest and abdomen a single block in thoracic duct does not cause chylothorax or chylous ascites.

LYMPHATICS OF HEAD AND NECK

The lymph nodes concerned in the drainage of head and neck remain mostly in neck. Out of 800 lymph nodes in body about 300 lymph nodes are present in neck, still more in children. Hence, neck is the organ that accommodates maximum lymph nodes. The lymph nodes are arranged both superficial and deep to the deep fascia (Fascia Colles) of neck.

Superficial Lymph Nodes

They are present superficial to the deep fascia of neck. They are arranged both transversely and longitudinally.

Transverse Nodes

- Submental nodes
- Submandibular nodes
- Postauricular nodes
- Preauricular nodes

- Superficial parotid nodes
- Buccal (Facial) nodes
- Occipital nodes.

Longitudinal Nodes

- Submental nodes
- Suprahyoid nodes
- Infrahyoid nodes
- Suprasternal nodes (in space of Burn)
- Superficial cervical nodes (These are present along the course of external jugular vein)
- Anterior cervical (present on the mid line of neck below hyoid bone).

Deep Lymph Nodes

The deep group of lymph nodes are arranged both anterior and posterior to sternocleidomastoid muscle, hence anterior and posterior group.

Anterior Deep Cervical Group

Upper set

a. Submandibular nodes
b. Jugulodigastric nodes
c. Sublingual nodes.

Lower set

a. Retropharyngeal nodes
b. Retrotracheal nodes
c. Paratracheal nodes.

Posterior Deep Cervical Group

Upper set

a. Suboccipital nodes
b. Jugular nodes (behind internal jugular vein)
c. Deep occipital nodes.

Lower set

a. Jugulo-omohyoid nodes
b. Supraclavicular nodes (on left known as Virchow's gland)
c. Subclavian nodes.

The filarial manifestation of cervical nodes is very rare. Hence, only the groups of lymph nodes are described in short in this chapter. The brain and spinal cord are devoid of lymphatic drainage for which filariasis is not manifest in this system.

CIRCULATION OF LYMPH

The lymphatic system is not provided with a pump as in circulation of blood. But it is still wonder the lymph circulates with same speed of blood. The factors responsible for circulation of lymph are:

Filtration Pressure

Due to constant generation of tissue fluid a pressure is created in the tissue space. This pressure forces the extra fluid with the end products of metabolism into the lymphatics opened into the tissue space.

Muscle Pump

Due to contraction of voluntary muscles the lymph in lymphatic channel is squeezed for forward movement thus a circulation is maintained.

Negative Intrathoracic Pressure

Due to negative intrathoracic pressure and positive intra-abdominal pressure the lymph is pushed from abdomen to thorax. This movement usually occurs in each movements of diaphragm.

Negative Neck Veins Pressure

The lymph always enters the blood circulation through the veins in the neck. The venous pressure in neck is always in negative side. Hence the lymph is sucked into veins in neck during diastole of right atrium.

Pulsation of Arteries

Because of arterial pulsation the lymphatics are pressed constantly leading to the movement of lymph.

The lymphatics are also provided with smooth muscles. This plays a very minor role in lymph flow.

chapter 2

Physiology of Tissue Circulation

Every cell needs nutrition for it is survival. The nutrition which comes from food reaches the blood circulation after digestion in gastrointestinal system. To reach at the tissue spaces the nutrients pass through arteries to veins in which the capillaries act the main passage to the tissue space. The pressure at arteriol side is 32 mm Hg and that at veniol side 16 mm Hg which has a tendency to push the plasma towards tissue space (see Fig. 2.1).

As the uncotic tension of plasma is 25 mm Hg which is due to presence of plasma proteins in blood has a tendency to draw tissue fluid towards the vascular channels. Therefore, the plasma enters the tissue space at the rate of 32 mm Hg—25 mm Hg (7 mm Hg) at arteriol side where as the tissue fluid enters the vascular channels at the rate of 25 mm Hg—16 mm Hg (9 mm Hg) at veniol side. Because of tissue fluid reaching the tissue space from vascular channels the nutrients present in blood easily reaches the tissue space. After metabolism the end products of the nutrients enter the vascular channel at veniol ends but the high molecular weight end products of the metabolism can not pass into the vascular channels. They pass into lymphatics and finally reaches the same blood circulation for its elimination either through kidneys or through skin. The plasma enters the tissue space at the force of (32–25) 7 mm Hg pressure at arteriol end but the tissue fluid enters the vascular channel at the force of (25–16) 9 mm Hg pressure at veniol end. This is because the end products of metabolism are more dangerous for tissue which needs easily removal and clearance from tissue producing it.

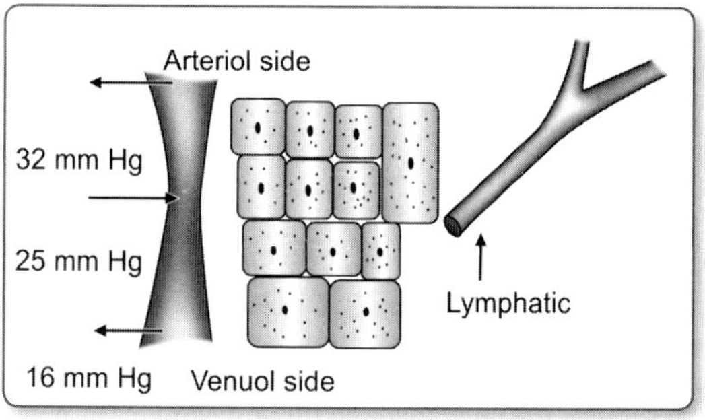

Fig. 2.1: Tissue space

Edema

The edema is a condition in which there is accumulation or collection of excessive tissue fluid in tissue space due to either excessive production or less or drainage of the tissue fluid. Edema prevents tissue oxygenation. (tissue hypoxia)

Classification of Edema

1. Low protein edema: When there is less of plasma protein persent particularly albumin in blood the uncotic tension becomes less (below 25 mm Hg) thereby more of plasma fluid enters the tissue space leading to edema. Normally the plasma enters the tissue space at arteriol side and returns do vascular channels at veniol side but due to low uncotic tension in hypoproteinemia the plasma also enters the tissue space at veniol end. What is known as reverse flow. Conditions leading to this type of edemas are seen in cirrhosis of liver, malignancies of liver (Hepatogenic), nephrotic syndrome, glomerulonephritis (Nephrogenic), congestive cardiac failure, Mitral and Tricuspid stenosis (cardiogenic) kwashiorkor disease low intake proteins (Nutritional) Anemia and hypoproteinemia (Hematogenic) Tuberculosis, leprosy (Infectious) and in all malignant conditions.

2. High protein edema.
   (a) High flow high protein edema: This condition mostly occurs in traumatic and surgical edema wherein there is leakage of blood into tissue space causing edema. Its an inflammatory edema following tissue reacting to trauma.
   (b) Low flow high protein edema: This type of edema occurs when there is blockage to lymphatic in case of filariasis and secondaries in lymph nodes lymphedema can be primary or secondary depending on its cause. Primary lymphedema may be present at birth but usually appears at after puberty. Some times this type of lymphedema does not manifest until old age. It is said that if there is no obvious cause for lymphedema arising in a patient above 30 years, "It is mostly due to malignancy unless and until prove to be otherwise."

       Secondary lymphedema is caused by either damage or removal of lymphatics following surgery or exposure to radiation. By far the most common cause of secondary lymphedema is due to filariasis. Chronic venous diseases always involves large lymhatics because they accompany the large veins. Thus lympedema is superimposed on venous edema making it a very bad condition like ulcers and gangrene leading to a condition called as "The safety valve edema".
3. Allergic edema: In this type of edema there is excessive liberation of histamin in tissue space due to allergic condition. Angioneurotic edema comes under this category.

chapter 3

Pathology of Filariasis

The filariasis is a disease of human being a result of infection caused by *Wuchereria bancrofti* and *Brugia malayi*. In addition to the above nematodes there may be other groups causing certain cutaneous filariasis such as *Loa loa* (Loiasis) and *Onchocerca volvulus* (Onchocerciasis). In this chapter the filariasis is explained in the light of *bancrofti* and *malayi* group lymphatic filariasis.

Distribution

Bancroftian filariasis is a disease widely spread in tropics and subtropics like America, West Indies, Argentine, Spain, Africa, India, China, Australia Middle East, etc. In India it is distributed usually in coastal zones like West Bengal, Orissa, Tamil Nadu, Maharashtra, Karnataka, Andhra Pradesh, Kerala as well as Gujarat. Other states like Bihar, Uttar Pradesh, Madhya Pradesh, etc. are not free from this disease.

The distribution of Malayan filariasis is mainly in India, Sri Lanka, Indonesia, Pakistan, Bangladesh, etc. Hence, in India both infections are usually found. Bancroftian filariasis is more towards northern India where as Malayan filariasis is more towards southern India. Mixed infections are also observed in Orissa.

Filariasis occupies about 2.5 to 3.8 percent of the total diseases in Orissa where as its incidence rate is average of 1 to 1.5 percent only. In order to transmit the disease it requires a vector such as mosquito.

Human being is the definite host whereas mosquito is the intermediate host for such disease. The adult worms mainly remain in the lymphatics and lymph nodes of human being only. This disease is not a Zoonotic disease (i.e. it does not affect other animals).

PARASITOLOGY

There are many filarial adult worms which are of different habits. Each of them prefers to remain in a particular tissue. A table is given below of the adult worms as per their tissue habits.

1. Lymphatic system
   — *Wuchereria bancroftl*
   — *Brugia malayi*
2. Connective tissue
   — *Onchocerca volvulus*
   — *Loa loa*
   — *Acanthocheilonema perstans*
   — *Mansonella ozzardi*
   — *Acanthocheilonema streptocerca*

The adult worms usually cause the pathological manifestation in human being and the microfilariae of the adult worms are also responsible for pathogenesis of the disease. The microfilariae of the different worms are found to have the habit as follows:

1. In blood
   — *Microfilariae bancrofti, Microfilariae malayi, Microfilariae loa*
   — *Microfilariae perstans* and *Microfilariae ozzardi,*
2. In skin
   — *Microfilariae volvulus, Microfilariae streptocerea*

In this chapter the life cycle of *Wuchereria bancrofti* and *Brugia malayi* are explained in details as filariasis usually means to the infections caused by these nematodes.

MORPHOLOGY

Wuchereria Bancrofti

Adult Worm

These are long hair like nematodes having one tappering end (tail side) and the headside is little rounded. This worm is transparent and bears no color at all. The male worm is short and less in number. The length of male worm measures about 3.5 to 4.0 cm, and 0.1 mm in thickness. The females worm is longer than males and abundant in number. 'The usual length of female adult worm is about 8 to 10 cm and thickness is about 0.2 to 0.3 mm. The female is ovoviviparous in type (i.e. it gives birth to ova inside which the embryo is located). The life- span is usually 4 to 5 years. The male worm is surrounded by many female worms for which it is difficult to see a male adult worm under microscope. The adult worms are only found in lymphatics and in lymph nodes. They never enter into blood circulation.

Microfilaria: The most active form of adult worm is this microfilaria or embryo. It can move both with and against blood stream. Like adult worm it is transparent and can remain in lymphatic system. They are produced in lymphatic system by the adult worms and enters the circulation through the main lymphatic trunks due to their active mobility. The embryo measures about 300 μ, in length and 10 μ in breadth. The embryo is surrounded by a tough membrane known as hyaline sheath in which space is provided for forward and backward movements of such embryo. There are many granules seen in the central axis of such microfilaria extending from head and to some part of the tail. This is called as somatic cells. These cells are found absent in about 5 percent of total length of the embryo in tail side. This is the characteristics of this bancroftian embryo. The somatic cells also lacking in head end side called cephalic space. In this embryo a nerve ring is provided nearer to the anterior end and both anus and other excretory pores, are also found in this microfilaria. The alimentary system of the embryo is called as central body of manson. Genital cells or "G" cells are usually one to four in number, and are arranged in chronological order for the purpose of reproduction.

Life cycle—*Wuchereria bancrofti* passes through two hosts in its life cycle like man and mosquito. The man is the definite host whereas mosquito is the intermediate host. In man the adult worms give birth to embryoes in lymphatic system from which they enter the circulation. This form of embryo can survive in circulation without undergoing any morphological changes. This embryo is taken by the mosquitoes during their blood meals, where the role of intermediate host comes to picture. For Bancroftian filariasis, *Culex fatigans* behaves as the intermediate host. Recently in a study it is observed that anopheles and aedes group of mosquitoes can act as intermediate hosts in addition to culex group. The female mosquitoes are mainly responsible for such spread of this disease. The microfilaria when taken by the mosquitoes undergoes morphological changes in alimentary canals of the mosquito, first hyaline sheath dissolves and microfilaria reduces in size. During this period microfilaria penetrates the stomach, migrates into the thoracic muscles. This larva is known as "First stage larva". After 3rd day of the ingestion the larva increases in size and cuticular cell vanishes resulting in "Second stage larva". After 10 to 12 days the larva, undergoes definite metamorphosis in which digestive, and genital system develop. This is known as "Third stage larva". This stage is infective stage for human being. The total duration for development of infective stage in mosquito is about two weeks. The third stage larva enters the proboscis of mosquito by help of which this can get its way to human body during bites. No sooner the larva penetrates the skin it finds its way into the lymphatic system where it grows to adult worm. An adult worm becomes sexually mature within 5 to 20 months time for production of microfilariae in lymphatic system in human body after which the microfilaria circulates in blood awaiting for, to be taken by mosquitoes in their blood meals.

Brugia Malayi

Adult worm—This nematode is long and hair like but shorter than *Wuchereria bancrofti*. It is colorless and transparent. The male worm is shorter than female worm. Like bancroftian worm the male worm is less in number. They usually remain in lymphatics and lymph nodes but the adult worms are not found in abdominal and inguinal group of lymph nodes. Hence, chances of chyluria and filariasis of scrotum are very much rare in malayan infection. The length of male is about 2 to 4 cm and thickness is about 0.1 mm. The length of female worm is 7 to 9 cm and thickness is 0.2 mm it is also ovoviviparous in nature. In all other respects it resembles that of *Wuchereria bancrofti.*

Microfilaria (Embryo)—The Microfilaria of *Brugia malayi* can survive both in lymphatics and blood circulation. It is produced by adult worms in lymphatic system but enters the blood circulation via main lymph trunk. Like bancroftian microfilaria, it can move both with and against the current of blood circulation. The microfilaria measures about 200 to 230 μ in length and thickness being 5 to 6 μ. The microfilaria is having multiple kinks. The outer layer of microfilaria is known as hyaline sheath in which a space is provided for to and fro movements of the embryo. The cephalic space is, wider than that of bancroftian microfilaria. Unlike bancroftian microfilaria the tail is provided with somatic cells. This is the characteristic feature of this microfilaria. There are two stylets, present at anterior end of this microfilaria as oppose to bancroftian type. All other features are like that of bancroftian microfilaria.

Life Cycle

Man is the definite host whereas mosquito is the intermediate host. Unlike bancroftian type mosquitoes of mansonoides and anopheles type act as intermediate host but never Culex group. The larva stage of mansonioidis group usually prefers to grow in water plants like pistia, Water-hyacinth and swamp grass. The life cycle of this microfilaria is same as bancroftian type but duration is about one week (6 to 7 days) whereas that in bancroftian microfilaria it is two weeks. Monkeys can act as definite host in addition to human being. Like bancroftian microfilaria the "3rd stage larva", is the infective stage of such microfilaria.

Periodicity

The bancroftian microfilaria usually appears in peripheral blood in between 10 pm and 4 am. During day time the microfilaria remains in the capillaries of lungs, kidneys, heart and other vital organs. In many countries it is found that this microfilaria found in peripheral circulation during day time. The exact cause of this periodicity is obscure till date but it can be explained that due to night habits of mosquito bites the microfilaria appears in peripheral blood at night for further spread. As aedes group bites during day time such microfilariae can be found in peripheral blood during day time. The malayan microfilariae can be seen in peripheral blood during day time because of mansonioidis behavior of biting during day time. Hence, the periodicity of microfilaria depends upon the time of bites of concerned mosquitoes responsible as the intermediate host in order to spread it to next host (Table 3.1).

PATHOGENESIS OF FILARIASIS

It is clear that the adult worms of filariasis remain in lymphatic system. Their main stay is in lymph nodes where they produce the microfilariae and enter the blood circulation via main lymphatic trunks. The microfilariae again enter the lymphatic system after getting sexually mature in blood circulation. They may also be taken by the intermediate hosts in order to complete the life cycle. Though the microfilariae remain in blood circulation, they are non-pathogenic as far as the disease is concerned. It is the adult worm that along with microfilariae in lymphatic system produce all symptomatology of this disease. The adult worms whether living or dead are equally responsible for pathogenesis of this disease.

An infected mosquito, when bites discharges the 3rd stage larva into the skin from where this infective form of larva gets its way into the local lymphatic channels. From this channel the larva reaches the

Table 3.1: Comparison between *W. bancrofti* and *B. malayi*.

	Wuchereria bancrofti	*Brugia malayi*
Adult Worms		
1. Habits	Lymphatics and all lymph nodes	Lymphatic systems except lymph nodes of abdomen and inguinal region
2. Length	Male—2.5 to 4 cm Female—8 to 10 cm	Male—2 to 4 cm Female—7 to 9 cm
Microfilaria		
1. Shape	Smooth curve	Multiple kinks
2. Size	$300 \times 10\ \mu$	$230 \times 5\ \mu$
3. Cephalic space	Long and broad	Short and broad
4. Tail	No somatic cell	Somatic cells present
5. Stylet	One	Two
Life Cycle		
1. Definite host	Man	Man and monkey
2. Intermediate host	Usually culex group (Anopheles and Aedes)	Usually manso-noidis group (Anopheles may be seen)
3. Period	Two weeks	One week
4. Infective stage	3rd stage larva	3rd stage larva
Periodicity	Usually night (from 10 pm to 4 am)	Usually day time

draining lymph node where this infective larva matures and becomes an adult worm. Similarly male and female adult worms conjugate for production of microfilariae. The injurious influence produced by the adult worms as well as microfilariae in the lymphatic system is an inflammatory reaction focussed in this system. This leads to either lymphadenitis or lymphangitis. These pathogenic effects are mainly due to mechanical obstruction as well as irritation by the adult worms during their movements inside the lymphatic system. The adult worms produce many metabolites during their metabolism. Some toxins (mainly endotoxin) are also produced by these adult worms. The metabolites as well as the toxins are highly irritant to the endothelial lining of the lymphatic system, thereby leads to lymphangitis or lymphadenitis. The female worms are capable of producing exotoxin during time of parturition. Due to absorption of these endo and exotoxins the patient first develops rigor with allergic fever before the development of lymphangitis or lymphadenitis. The damage to the endothelial layer of lymphatic system invites bacterial infection caused by streptococci mainly. Hence, the duration of fever depends upon severity of bacterial infection as well as liberation of toxins. Because of local edema of lymph nodes and lymphatics due to inflammation and infection the concerned lymph node becomes palpably tender. As the capsule of the lymph node is non-stretchable but sensitive, a constant pain is felt due to increased tension inside the capsule. The lymph nodes and lymphatic channels are obliterated due to the following reasons like in early stage.

a. Mechanical obstruction caused by bolus of adult worms and microfilariae.
b. Edema of lymphatic system caused by inflammation as well as bacterial infection.
c. Proliferation of endothelium is response to toxic inflammation.

As soon as the lymph nodes and lymphatics become edematous the draining area is deprived of lymphatic drainage. This leads to local edema due to local collection of lymph. This lymph is in fluid state, hence it always collects in the dependent part and in parts easy to accommodate the fluid. For these reasons the lymph edema in early stage is pitting. The lymph collects in subcutaneous space as the skin is stretchable but lymph rarely collects inside the muscular compartment due to presence of deep fascia which is non-elastic. The contraction of muscles prevents the collection of lymph inside muscle compartments. The organs involved during this process will present according to its function. This edema will increase in size if untreated and local infections by streptococci and staphylococci is mandatory. The lymph is rich in carbohydrate as well as protein, which helps in growth of microorganisms. Due to local infection, cellulitis occurs in the affected part. As soon as the body immunity comes to play a part, this infection becomes localized and leads to abscess formation or ulceration of the part. Depending upon the previous condition of the patient the cellulitis can spread to the end in gangrene or septicemia as well. If in this stage proper antibiotics are started the lymphatic system becomes free of obstruction thereby all symptoms subside automatically. The cellulitis of the part can subside automatically if the immunity is strong enough or early treatment started by proper antibiotics and antihistamine. Due to liberation of allergens by adult worms the total eosinophilic count may increase but neutrophiles can show hyperactivity due to local infection. In late stage of this disease plasma cells and lymphocytes may increase in number in order to increase the antibodies against filariasis.

Involvement of lymphatics of retroperitoneal space and septicemia can invite paralytic ileus for which distension of abdomen and vomiting are possible during each acute attacks. Pylorospasm is seen when the infection is localized to abdominal lymphatics which indicates that lymphatics of stomach are directly connected with lymphatics of abdomen. Hence, it can be said "stomach is the loudspeaker of abdomen".

In late stage of this disease fibrosis develops surrounding lymphatics and in lymph nodes. This causes complete obstruction of lymphatic channels and further development of lymphedema. Due to repeated infections there is local fibrosis and coagulation of lymph proteins. This condition resembles like the skin of an elephant hence elephantiasis. The edema in late state becomes non-pitting. The distal lymphatic channels may dilate leading to a condition called lymphangiectasis or lymph varix. The dilated lymphatic channels can rupture causing chyluria, lymphorrhea, chylothorax, chylocele, chylous ascites or chylous diarrhea in respect to sight and organs involved. In an elephantial organ if a superficial infection begins (usually fungal) the ulcer persists constantly because of heavy fibrosis which prevents epithelization. The infection is difficult to eradicate as the edematous part is, rich in culture media and fibrosis also partly responsible for persistence of infection. A fibrotic lymph node can undergo calcification due to repeated infections. Organ like testis undergoes calcification for such reasons. It will not be out of place to emphasis that immunity plays a major role in this disease. The reticulo-endothelial system of lymph nodes is directly involved by this disease. If the immunity is strong enough the patient may not suffer from acute manifestation of filariasis in which edema may be seen without local signs of infection. The deep lymphangitis and perineural lymphangitis may present like polyneuritis in filariasis. Microfilariae have been cultured from blood, hydrocele fluid, chyles and aqueous humorous of eyeballs.

Histopathology

The adult worm of filariasis is more responsible for histopathological changes in lymphatic system than the microfilariae. The changes are invited by a dead worm than a living worm. An adult worm when dead, liberates all toxins into the lymphatic system. Many authors believe that the movements of microfilariae and adult worms in lymphatic system are responsible for such histological changes.

As the reticuloendothelial system is located in lymph nodes, an immunological change is marked in lymphatic system at an early date. Liberation of toxins by adult worms, the endothelial linings of lymphatics and lymph nodes undergo reactionary proliferation. There is eosinophilic infiltration to the substance of lymph nodes and thereby stroma of lymphatic system becomes edematous. The edema and endothelial proliferation produce obstruction in the lymphatic channels thereby the adult worms are deprived of nutrition. The adult worms and microfilariae mainly survive by lymph only. Hence when there is obstruction to lymph flow, the adult worms become dead and undergo fragmentation and disintegration. A dead worm is more pathogenic to lymph nodes than a living worm.

As soon as bacterial infection supervenes there will be perivascular infiltration of polymorphonuclear cells, histocytes, lymphocytes, epithelioid cells and giant cells. Neovascularization is also marked in the infected lymph nodes. The giant cells and epithelioid cells are found surrounding the dead worms. No sooner the active infection subsides, granulomatous tissue accumulates in the diseased lymph nodes and perilymphatic fibrosis becomes prominent. Calcification of a lymph node is the last manifestation of this disease. Hence it is said "A calcified lymph node is a tombstone erected in the memory of filarial worms embedded inside it". A lymph node when calcified can be visualized by X-rays. The organs involved in filariasis show some histological changes. Edema of tissue is marked in early stage. The lymphatics and veins dilate and proliferate. There will be eosinophilic infiltration. Skin becomes hypertrophy and undergoes hyperkeratinization. The connective tissue and fatty tissue become edematous and local infiltration with round cells (like plasma cells and lymphocytes) and eosinophils is marked. The microfilariae or adult worms are very rarely seen in the affected organ. The muscle and bone rarely show any change. The muscles in early stage become hypertrophy but in late stage muscles show atrophic changes due to non-use.

PANI'S GRADATION OF EDEMA

For better clinical appreciation the lymph edema of the limbs is subjected to gradations. This gradation was implemented first in the filaria clinic at ESI Cottage hospital, Choudwar. The gradation of edema is done for better follow-up of the patients and their response to the treatment. The following points are taken into consideration for gradation of lymphedema of limbs.

a. Type of edema—Whether pitting or non-pitting or partially pitting.
b. Bony points—The bony points like medial malleolus, lateral malleolus, sin of tibia, tuberosity of calcaneum, styloid process of ulna, radial tuberosity, radial styloid process, olecronon-process of ulna, medial and lateral epicondyles of humerus, etc.
c. Condition of skin—Whether skin is healthy or unhealthy like ulceration, cellulitis, fungal infection, over granulation, lymphorrhea, etc.

GRADES OF EDEMA

Grade I

a. Edema is pitting
b. Bony points are not obliterated
c. Skin is healthy.

Grade II

a. Edema is pitting
b. Bony points are obliterated
c. Skin is healthy.

Grade III

a. Edema is partially or non-pitting (Fig. 3.1, Plate 1)
b. Bony points are obliterated
c. Skin is healthy.

Grade IV

a. Edema is non-pitting (Fig. 3.2, Plate 1)
b. Bony points are obliterated
c. Skin is unhealthy.

The gradation of limb edema bears some clinical importance. Usually grade I and grade II edema can subside with proper medical treatment, whereas grade III and grade IV edema require surgical intervention for its cure. Regarding scrotal and penile edema, gradation bears no clinical importance at all.

IMMUNOLOGY IN FILARIASIS

Acknowledgment

By: Prof Tribhuban Mohan Mohapatra, Division of Parasitology, Department of Microbiology, Institute of Medical Sciences, Banaras Hindu University, Varanasi-221005 (India).

Introduction

Filariasis is a disease of high endemicity in tropical zones affecting nearly 300 millions of people all over the world. This tropical disease produces wide spectrum of symptoms such as recurrent fever, lymphangitis, lymphadenitis, hydrocele of TVT, chyluria, tropical pulmonary eosinophilia, etc. Some individuals show no symptoms at all. Repeated exposure of individuals to filariasis fails to induce protective immunity, but leads to sub-clinical infections.

The cell mediated immunity status was measured by blast transformation of lymphocytes by using mitogen, phytohemagglutinin and D-immitis antigen (Dirofilaria immitis). In absence of the specific antigen D-immitis was used because within the antigenic mosaic of this nematode there exists a large number of factions which are common to all filarial species. T-cell status was assessed by E rosetting. Hypersensitivity reactions of the individuals to filarial antigens was studied by intradermal injections of D-immitis antigen.

The results of the filarial patients were compared with those of the normal healthy individuals residing in this area which is an endemic zone for Bancroftian-Filariasis.

IMMUNOPATHOGENESIS

Analysis of blastogenic response of various clinical categories of filariasis and controls to mitogenic and antigenic stimuli shows that asymptomatic microfilaria carriers and untreated filariasis patients exhibited significant cellular unresponsiveness. The treated patients also showed a significant reduction in the lymphocyte activity as compared to controls but they had an apparently improved cellular response. It is observed that immune response in clinical filariasis is depressed even to mitogenic stimuli. The mechanism of unresponsiveness is not clearly understood. The serum suppressor factors which are yet to be clearly defined has been suggested to depress the cell mediated immune (CMI) in filariasis. It is thought that immune suppression in filariasis is neither due to universal hormonal factor nor due to adherent cells. It may be due to suppression of host immune system by the microfilariae. The lymphocytic response was found to be most vigorous in endemic carriers. In an active filarial infection the lymphocytic response is highly depressed. Lymphatic leucocytosis along with significantly low percentage of E-rosette forming cells were observed in microfilaria carriers and patients, though the percentage of rosette forming cells were found to be increased in treated cases. T-cells lymphopenia may be due to transient relocation of lymphocyte pool, certain lymphocytotoxin, loss of specific T-cell subclass or serum inhibitory factors interfering with rosette formation in filariasis. It may be interesting to speculate whether the loss of T-lymphocytes in the filariasis patients represent the deletion of clones, previously committed to respond to the filarial antigens which resulted in cellular unresponsiveness. No hypersensitivity reaction is observed to D-immitis antigen in endemic cases but in case of filarial carriers and acute filarial infection the reaction of skin D-immitis antigen is very much hypersensitive. The role of diethyl carbamazine citrate (DEC) in modifying the immediate hypersensitivity reaction in filarial patients is well known because of it is weak antihistaminic property.

IMMUNODIAGNOSIS OF FILARIASIS

The sensitivity and specificity of the enzyme linked immuno-sorbent-Assay (ELISA) the indirect hem agglutination (IHA) test and the countercurrent immunoelectrophoresis (CIEP) test were assessed in the diagnosis of filariasis. Positive reactions were observed in 91 per-cent and 86 percent of cases by ELISA and IHA tests respectively. CIEP test detected only 31.5 percent of cases. Cross reaction due to intestinal helminthiasis was observed in 80 percent of cases by both in ELISA and IHA test whereas with CIEP cross reaction was observed in 10 percent of cases. The microfilaria count was inversely proportional to the antibody titre among asymptomatic carriers ELISA was the most sensitive test followed by IHA and then CIEP. The CIEP test though it detected only a small number of cases, was observed to be the most specific.

Lyophilized saline extract of Dirofilaria immitis (D-immitis) is used as a source of antigen for the serological tests in filariasis. Five millilitres of blood (venous) is required for collection of serum to be used at 20°C with addition 1:1000 sodium azide for further test.

It is concluded that for the diagnosis these serological tests clearly show their advantage over the conventional parasitological examination. The concentration technique which can detect even low levels of parasitemia can hardly be applied for diagnosis of and epidemiological studies due to its technical difficulties. Use of D-immitis antigen for serological method represents a suitable alternative for the diagnosis of filaria cases and asymptomatic microfilaria carriers.

Classification of Filariasis in Clinical Practice

chapter 4

Acute Presentations

Acute filarial fever, acute lymphangitis, acute lymphadenitis, acute orchitis, acute epididymo-orchitis, acute funiculitis, acute mastitis, acute salpingitis, acute oophoritis, acute arthritis, acute synovitis, acute myositis, acute tendinitis, acute urinary tract infection, acute retroperitonial lymphangitis, cellulities, abscess, ulcers and gangrene.

Chronic Presentations

Lymphatic Block with Distal Dilatation

— Lymphangiectasis (Lymph Varix)
— Hydrocele of scrotum (Lymph Scrotum)
— Hydrocele of breast.

Lymphatic Block with Distal Dilatation and Rupture

— Chyluria, chylothorax, chylous diarrhea, chylocele, chylous ascites and lymphorrhea.

Lymphatic Block with Lymph Stasis

Elephantiasis of upper limb and lower limb, elephantiasis of breast.

Elephantiasis of scrotum with or without Ram-horn penis, Elephantiasis of vulva.

Silent Presentation

— Hydrocele of TVT
— Tropical eosinophilia
— Angioneurotic edema.

Acute Presentations of Filariasis

chapter 5

ACUTE FILARIAL FEVER

Clinical Features

The incubation period for filariasis is about one year as the 3rd stage larva takes about one year to mature to be all adult worm. It is already clear that adult worms are responsible for pathogenesis of filariasis. Due to such a prolonged incubation period, the children below 2 years, never suffer from filariasis. The filariasis is very rare in children below ten years. The microfilariae cannot pass through the blood-brain barrier as well as placental barrier. Hence, congenital filarial manifestation is not observed in clinical practice. This disease is equally distributed in adult and no age above two years is immune to this disease. The filariasis is more in males than in females. In a recent study at ESI Cottage Hospital, Choudwar, it is found that this disease is more amongst females in industrial belts. However, sex bears no relation with filariasis.

The filarial fever begins with rigor and tremor throughout body. This comes with sudden onset and persists nearly one to three hours. The patient feels cold and shivery throughout the body but it is more marked in extremities and back. There may be flushing of face and conjunctival congestion. The mucous membrane of pharynx, larynx and nose are congested and lacrimation with nasal discharge are marked at this stage. This is due to toxin and allergens produced by microfilariae and adult worms. The heart rate or pulse rate is markedly increased in this stage due to stress and strain but in some patients it is observed, the pulse rate may remain normal or less due to low body temperature. Some patients complain of palpitation during rigor stage of filariasis. The temperature becomes subnormal (96 or 97°F) in the beginning of rigor stage. The patient demands heavy covers by thick blankets and feels better after pressure over his back. Some patients vomit during or before onset of rigor if they had heavy meals on the same day. This vomiting is more marked in patients who suffer from inguinal or abdominal lymphadenitis. The vomiting may continue for two to three days due to onset of gastritis constipation and distension of abdomen are common features in filariasis. The patient is conscious throughout the attack as filariasis never affects central nervous system due to absence of lymphatics in this system. The rigor shows its severity in patients, having low vitality, in patients of diabetes, first attack of filariasis, anemia and hypertension. The rigor indicates heavy production of histamine and H-like substances in response to liberation of toxins and allergens by dead adult worms. The severity of rigor depends upon production of histamines and H-like substances with liberation of natural antihistamines like glucocorticoid and catecholamines (Adrenaline and Nor-adrenaline). In some patients rigor may not appear and local manifestation will be the only sign in filariasis.

As soon as rigor subsides, fever supervenes. The patient develops headache and bodyache. The temperature varies from 100 to 104°F. Normally this fever continues for 2 to 3 days. The fever is of continuous type and may be lowered in early morning. In some patients it is observed that the temperature becomes normal in morning but rises at evening. The double rise in temperature is seen in some patients of filariasis. The pulse rate and respiration rate increase during fever stage. The pulse rate rises by 10 in each rise of 1°F of temperature. The tongue is coated and the breath is foul smelling. There may be cough with or without expectoration due to bronchitis. This bronchitis is mainly due to tropical eosinophilia. Ronchi and crepitation may be present in some patients, distension of abdomen and sluggishness of bowel sound is usually marked in this time. Epigastric tenderness can be elicited in filariasis due to gastritis. Constipation is an usual feature in fever stage of filariasis. Conjunctival congestion and flushing of face are well marked in fever-stage of filariasis. Some patients complain of burning pain in micturition and pain in joints and in muscles. Due to secondary streptococcal infection in lymphatics, septicemia is the dominating feature in the entire show. Dehydration is also seen in this stage due to vomiting and loss of fluid in insensible perspiration, nausea and anorexia are common during entire period of filarial fever. The rigor and fever bear no relation with number of attacks of acute filariasis. The fever comes in each 15 to 30 days interval and in some patient it is marked in a particular day of each month. The fever when subsides the local sign of filariasis come to light and concerned group of lymph nodes become painful and tender. There may be edema of the concerned limb or organ.

The hematological picture in filariasis is increased in eosinophilic count and neutrophilic count. The eosinophilia is found in 5 to 15 percent of cases. The neutrophilia is due to bacterial infection and septicemia. The lymphocytosis is found in chronic patients of filariasis where eosinophilia is absent. The microfilariae can be seen in night blood of the patient. The microfilariae are not found in peripheral blood in chronic cases like elephantiasis, in early allergic manifestation and after acute attack of lymphangitis due to death of the adult worms. The intradermal test for allergic manifestation and compliment fixation test, though advocated in filariasis are not reliable for diagnosis of filariasis. Biopsy of concerned lymph node and affected tissue will confirm the diagnosis but it is not possible to do the biopsy in all cases. The clinical and hematological diagnosis is more dependable than histopathological diagnosis.

Differential Diagnosis

There are many febrile conditions which mimic filariasis. These are known as elephantoid fever such as.

Malaria

Normally malarial fever has three stages of events such as rigor, fever and sweating. Usually total duration is about one to three hours. The sweating is not found in filariasis and fever is continuous. Spleen and liver are usually palpable in malaria whereas such are not marked in filarial fever. The patient becomes afebrile in between attacks of malaria whereas the temperature rarely touches the base line in filariasis. The malarial parasites (BT and MT rings) are seen in red-blood cells during the attack of fever whereas microfilariae are not found during filarial attacks.

Subphrenic Abscess

"Pus somewhere, pus nowhere else pus under the diaphragm". Pain in abdomen more in right hypochondrium, hiccough, rigor with hectic rise in temperature and sweating are features of subphrenic abscess. Tender and enlarged (due to displacement) liver is also seen in this condition, whereas liver is normal in filariasis. Radiological findings confirm the diagnosis in subphrenic abscess.

Enteric Fever

The typhoid fever is an infectious disease characterized by continuous fever, discomfort or pain in abdomen, enlarged spleen, (Liver at times) relative bradycardia, rose spots eruption of skin, leucopenia with relative lymphocytosis. Leucopenia, bradycardia and enlarged spleen are not found in filariasis. Local signs of lymphatic involvement is not seen in typhoid fever.

Treatment

As the filarial fever is mainly caused by a toxin and allergens produced by adult worm and super added by streptococcal infection, the antibiotics and antihistamines are the drug of choice in early stage.

Antifilarial drugs are not given in acute stage as the same will aggravate the condition. Vitamins and hematinics are given in order to support the immunological system of the body.

Antibiotics like penicillin, streptomycin, sulpha group and tetracycline are of choice. Many surgeons do not agree with streptomycin as this antibiotic produces perilymphatic fibrosis which helps in filarial edema, as soon as the acuteness subsides, antifilarial drugs are to be given (see chapter on Antifilarial Drugs).

LYMPHADENITIS AND LYMPHANGITIS

Clinical Features

The lymphadenitis and lymphangitis are complimentary to each other. Whenever there is lymphadenitis there is always some amount of lymphangitis, but this may not be clinically detected. Whereas whenever there is lymphangitis there must be draining lymph nodes infection.

Commonly lymph nodes of inguinal, axillary epitrochlear, popliteal and abdominal regions are involved in filariasis. The lymphatics of lower limb and upper limb are involved in filariasis in order of merit. The major portions of lymphatics of skin, drain either to inguinal or axillary group of lymph nodes for which involvement of these lymph nodes in filariasis is common. The lymphadenitis and lymphangitis can present per se or this may be a part of acute filarial fever.

As in acute filarial fever this presents as pain, fever and local signs of involvement of lymph nodes are in order of sequence. The patients complain of pain in a localized area of involvement and followed by acute filarial fever. As soon as local signs develop the fever subsides gradually due to localization of the disease. In acute lymphadenitis or lymphangitis there may not be typical acute filarial fever but in such cases careful history taking will reveal presence of bodyache, headache and rise in temperature up to 99 to 100°F. This may continue for 2 to 3 days. Past history of repeated attacks of lymphadenitis or lymphangitis may be present in such cases.

In case of lymphadenitis the lymph nodes are enlarge and tender on palpation. The lymph nodes retain their shape and size in early stage but such appearance disappears when the lymph nodes become edematous. In early attacks the lymph nodes are discrete and mobile as the infection is centrally placed. In prolonged and chronic cases the lymph nodes may undergo matting due to involvement of capsules by the process of infection. There may be edema of surrounding tissue and skin. The skin may be red congested and pitting edema can be demonstrated. In this stage the lymph nodes may become normal due to early treatment or development of immunity. In non-treated cases there can be abscess formation and death of covering skin. When the abscess ruptures it will lead to sinus formation and ulceration. The lymph nodes loose their shape and size permanently if involved once by abscess formation. Persistence of sinus and ulcer indicates presence of deep seated slough and other foreign substance in that area. Repeated attacks of acute lymphadenitis become chronic in nature and this helps the lymph node to undergo calcification. The calcified lymph nodes cast shadow by X-rays like irregular mottled appearance and calcification is more in periphery than in center. A lymph node when calcified rarely gets next chance of streptococcal reinfection. Hence, calcification indicates a healed lesion of an old infection.

In case of iliac lymphadenitis patients complain of pain in iliac fossa and such in right side mimics the picture of appendicitis. There may be fixed flexion deformity of the hip joint due to spasm of ileo-psoas muscles. The mass is fixed to the pelvic wall in which fingers cannot be inserted between mass and pelvic wall. Untreated cases may present as iliac abscess which requires drainage through extraperitonial route.

In case of lymphangltls the llmbs are common sltes of Involvement. Usually the draining lymph nodes show some amount of infection. Acute filarial fever can be a warning sign in lymphangitis. There will be an elongated cord like swelling on the long axis of the limb. Edema of the surrounding tissue and tenderness are usual signs. Normally the skin is adherent to this swelling. The color of the swelling is red which is well marked in white colored patients. The swelling is firm in consistency and beaded. Some patients complain of burning pain and numbness along the swelling due to involvement of cutaneous nerves. The movement of limb is painful if the swelling is adherent to the surrounding muscles. Normally, the medial side of upper limb and lower limb are site of involvement of such disease. The swelling can move on the transverse axis but not on the longitudinal axis.

When a vein is involved by this process thrombophlebitis is seen in this vein. Untreated case can show abscess formation and ulceration. The chronic and old cases can undergo calcification. Lymphorrhea and lymph varix are seen on the involved skin which invites fungal infections very soon. Scaling of skin is marked when such lesion heals and ulceration is also possible in some cases.

Differential Diagnosis

Tuberculous Lymphadenitis

Normally the lymph nodes of neck are the site of tuberculosis whereas filariasis affects inguinal and axillary lymph nodes commonly. Central caseation with early matting are seen in tuberculosis whereas such are the findings in late cases of filariasis. Pain and tenderness are usually absent in tuberculosis due to chronicity of this disease unless superadded with secondary infection. Histopathological study confirms the diagnosis in both conditions.

Syphilitic Lymphadenitis

In syphilis, the lymph nodes are involved either in primary stage or tertiary stage. The lymph nodes are discrete, mobile, soft in consistency (shotty) painless and slightly tender. In primary syphilis there will be primary sore along with enlargement of lymph nodes. Primary syphilis affects the inguinal lymph nodes whereas tertiary syphilis affect the epitrochlear and occipital lymph nodes. Serological test like VDRL and WR tests are positive after 10 days of primary infection.

Lymphogranuloma Venerium

It is a veneral disease caused by a filterable virus of psittacosis-lymphogranuloma inguinale group. In secondary lesion the lymph nodes of inguinal group are involved in this disease but it can spread to iliac group of lymph nodes in late cases. The lymph nodes enlarge but not mobile as early matting is possible due to periadenitis. The lymph nodes undergo central liquefaction and the overlying skin become adherent to it. If untreated, sinus formation and ulceration are the terminal result of such a disease. In females pararectal involvement causes rectal stricture. Freis intradermal test becomes positive in this disease.

Nonspecific Lymphadenitis

This commonly found in persons who walk in bare-foot. The lymph nodes are enlarged, firm in consistency, mobile or matted in late cases but nontender. It is very difficult to differentiate it from filariasis as the inguinal group is common site of this disease. Histopathological study shows all pictures of chronic bacterial infection without adult worms of filariasis.

Treatment

Like acute filarial fever antibiotics, antihistamines, vitamins and hematinics are the early treatment of choice in acute cases. As soon as acuteness sub-sides, antifilarial drugs are to be given to the patient. (See chapter on antifilarial drugs).

In order to correct the fixed flexion deformity of iliac lymphadenitis the patient should be subjected to traction of the lower limb for 2 to

3 weeks. In some cases it may be required to prolong the traction till the deformity is corrected.

In repeated infection the lymph nodes may be removed if swelling does not respond to the antifilarial treatment for continuously three months. Normally, the inguinal group may be required for such surgical removal. The mass should be subjected to biopsy. Care should be taken to avoid injury to vital structures in femoral region like femoral vein, artery and nerve. A drain is left for 24 to 48 hours in the wound to avoid hematoma.

ACUTE ORCHITIS, ACUTE EPIDIDYMITIS AND ACUTE FUNICULITIS

Clinical Features

The inflammation infection of testis epididymis and spermatic cord are known as orchitis, epididymitis and funiculitis respectively. Normally infection of one organ invites infection of other as the three organs are provided with single group of lymphatics and lymph nodes. Filariasis of genital organs in males occupies the second position in the list next to filariasis of lower limb but in females filarial mastitis is second to filariasis of limbs.

These patients complain commonly of pain with or without acute filarial fever. Unilateral involvement is usually seen in many cases. Usually one side is manifested first and subsequently other side can be involved in the same attack. Pain begins from the spermatic cord and spreads to both directions resulting involvement of epididymis and testis. The pain is continuous and dragging in nature. The testicular pain is usually referred to back as far as lumbar region as the testis has descended from abdomen to scrotum. "Brown's Law—Pain, produced in an organ which has migrated from its primary position, and which has not acquired an additional nerve supply in its secondary or permanent position, is invariably localized in the primary relative position of that organ". Some patients complain of pain as high as scapular region. This pain is exaggerated by movements or touch of testes and scrotum so much so that the patients cannot stand straight. The patients get relief of pain by support of the testis for which the patient holds his testes by his own hands during standing and walking (Prehn's sign). In order to avoid touch of scrotum to thighs the patient walks in position of abduction of thighs with support of scrotum by their own hands. There may be lumbar scoliosis and kyphosis. There may be features of acute filarial fever but typical filarial fever may not be present in all cases. However, such cases show some rise in temperature. Some patients complain of pain in abdomen particularly in iliac fossa, lumbar region and hypogastium due to involvements of iliac and para aortic lymph nodes. Distension of abdomen, constipation and vomiting may be present at the beginning of this disease. In severe cases, features of septicemia are marked. On examination of genital organs, there may be swelling of scrotum and testis with congestion. The scrotal veins may be dilated. The skin is elongated and pendulous due to increased volume of testis. The testis, epideymis and spermatic cord are tender and edematous. Testicular sensation is exaggerated in some cases and preserved very well. Hydrocele of tunica vaginalis testis is evident due to lack of absorption of such fluid. The sac may be thickened. Thickening of epididymis and spermatic cord are marked and tenderness is elecited during palpation. The vas may be thickened and beaded. Due to repeated attacks, epididymis and spermatic cord become irregular and fibrotic. In untreated cases, the fluid in tunica vaginalis testis may increase in amount and due to secondary infection by streptococci, staphylococci, and *E. coli*, changes the hydrocele to pyocele. The patients complain of constant throbbing type of pain in pyocele cases and the patients cannot sleep during this stage. There may be hectic rise in temperature with feature of septicemia. Minor trauma during this attack can produce hematocele of tunica vaginalis testis. Tenderness in iliac fossa and in abdomen is expected in all cases due to involvement of lymph nodes. Prolonged and repeated attacks of filarial orchitis help in calcification of tunica vaginalis testis which can cast shadow on radiological examination. In addition to iliac and para-aortic group, inguinal lymph nodes may be enlarged and tender. Trans-illumination test for hydrocele of tunica vaginalis testis may be positive in acute cases but this becomes negative when the fluid is blood (hematocele) or chyle (chylocele) or the sac is thickened. The size of the hydrocele increases in each attack of filariasis. As soon as the inguinal group of lymph nodes are involved the scrotum, penis and lower limb show features of filariasis.

The hematological picture is similar to acute filarial fever in which microfilariae can be isolated and lymph node biopsy can confirm the diagnosis.

Differential Diagnosis

Torsion of Testis

An anatomically normal testis is immune for torsion but only abnormally disposed testis is subjected for torsion. Torsion of one side is a guide for the involvement of opposite testis by the same process. Hence, contralateral testis should be subjected for treatment as soon as possible (even at the same time) in order to prevent its torsion. The patients are within the age of fifteen to twenty five but children can suffer from such disease. The torsion is centrifugal from the septum of scrotum. Prehn's sign is positive in all case of torsion, i.e. support of testis exaggerates the pain in torsion whereas in orchitis pain gets relief after support. Sudden onset of pain being referred to abdomen and vomiting without fever in a patient within twenty-five years of age, suspects the diagnosis of torsion than acute orchitis. Examination of opposite testis will reveal the anatomical abnormality in it. Untreated cases undergo gangrenous change due to lack of vascularity.

Traumatic Orchitis

In orchitis following trauma the patients complain of pain and swelling without acute onset of fever. There may be reactionary hydrocele or post-traumatic hematocele which can be diagnosed after transillumination test. Involvements of lymph nodes occur after secondary infection and fever is possible in this stage. Trauma of any degree can manifest a latent filariasis in genital organ. However, it is difficult to differentiate between filarial orchitis from traumatic orchitis clinically except taking the help of hematological investigations.

Tubercular Epididymitis

This is a painless and chronic process brought to the notice after minor injury or in course of examination. There may be slight pain in testis. Involvement of globus major indicates the disease is blood- born whereas such in globus minor indicates urogenital spread which is very common. The epididymis is nodular, discrete and irregular. The nodules may be slightly tender. The testis is normal and the testicular sensation is preserved till it becomes atrophic due to fibrosis following slow avascular necrosis. There may be lax secondary hydrocele in 30 per cent cases. The vas may be beaded which indicates that this is involved by tuberculous process being spread from above. In 20 per-cent cases there may be a discharging sinus from posterior surface of testis due to rupture of a cold abscess. In per rectal examination, the seminal vesicles as well as the prostate may be beaded and nodular. The seminal vesicles may be thickened and irregular. In such cases the epididymis may undergo calcification. Seminal and prostatic fluid analysis will reveal the presence of mycobacterium tuberculosis.

Syphilitic Orchitis

The syphilis attacks the body of the testis without involvement of epididymis. In congenital type bilateral orchitis is common but in acquired type unilateral manifestation is seen. The testis becomes atrophic due to interstitial fibrosis or it may increase in size in gummatous lesion. The testicular sensation is absent from the early manifestation of syphilitic orchitis. In gummatous lesion the testis enlarges and hard in consistency. There may be lax secondary hydrocele. The testis may be adherent to skin in late cases. The serological tests are strongly positive in syphilitic orchitis.

Tumors of Testis

The most common neoplasms of testis are seminoma manifests after 40 years whereas teratoma occurs before 40 years of age. In typical cases pain is a late feature unless there is metastasis. Seminoma spreads by lymphatics where as teratoma spreads by blood for which lungs and brain are the site of deposit. The testis enlarges uniformly in seminoma but irregular in teratoma. The testicular sensation becomes completely absent in late stage of neoplasm. The spermatic cord may be thickened in late cases due to hypertrophy of cremaster and increase paminiform plexus but vas remains normal throughout. There may be lax secondary hydrocele. Some cases may present like epididymo-orchitis but it does not respond to any antibiotic. Hence, it is said "failure to respond to a short sharp course of antibiotics in epididymo-orchitis it may be a tumor, unless proved to be otherwise". Excisional biopsy confirms the diagnosis.

Treatment

General Treatment

Like acute filarial fever antibiotics, antihistamines, vitamins and hematinics are the treatment of choice in early stage. As soon as the acuteness subsides antifilarial drugs should be given to the patient with an advice to come for regular check up till he is free from such disease at least for two years. All preventive measures are to be taken against the reinfection. Alkalization of urine may be an adjuvant therapy. The general treatment and local treatment should go hand in hand.

Local Treatment

In order to reduce pain scrotal support in any form, is vital in local treatment. Scrotal bandage or a suspensory bandage should be applied in early case of orchitis. Some surgeons prefer to give strapping between two thighs with cotton pad in between scrotum strapping. This support should be advised during resting period only.

The scrotal support, in any form, is essential till the patient is free from acuteness. This support not only relieves pain by reducing congestion but prevents complications like hydrocele, pyocele, hematocele, calcification and atrophy of testis. The support should not be too tight to produce pain or too loose to be useless in preventing complications. It is observed that people using tight underwears suffer less from hydrocele of tunica vaginalis testis and its complication.

When there is inflammatory effusion to the tunica vaginalis testis, the pyocele should be prevented by appropriate antibiotics and scrotal support. Some surgeons advocate needle aspiration in such cases under antibiotic cover. The aspiration of fluid from tunica vaginalis testis not only prevents the pyocele formation but also reduces the intrascrotal pressure thereby the atrophy of the testis is prevented. Care must be taken to prevent puncture of testis or any blood vessels of tunica vaginalis testis. Iatrogenic hematocele is only complication of needle aspiration. The local circulation increases after needle aspiration due to reduced intrascrotal pressure and this helps in early repair of damaged testis. The patient may require one to two aspirations in each attack. This aspiration should be done in full aseptic condition and by an experience surgeon. The needle should be inserted into the tunica vaginalis testis from anterolateral surface of the swelling. The testis should be palpated for its position before inserting the needle. In case of pyocele, the pus should be drained out as soon as possible and as far as practicable. This procedure is carried out under antibiotic umbrella. A small incision is to be given on the anterior surface of the scrotum as dependent as possible under local anesthesia. The tunica vaginalis testis is exposed and a puncture is to be made under direct vision. As soon as pus is drained out, one should palpate the testis to know its condition. If the testis is normal a gauge or globes drain is inserted inside the tunica vaginalis. Excision of sac is advised as soon as the test is free from infection, or condition of the patient is good to stand the operation in one stage. Some surgeons advocate the excision of sac or testis after three months but such a guideline is not advisable as repetition of such attack is possible within this period. One stage orchidectomy may be done if the testis is completely damaged and the contralateral testis is normal. During orchidectomy age and marital condition of the patient should be taken into consideration. "Tissue respect" is always kept in mind in orchidectomy operation.

The orchidectomy is indicated in pyocele (where testis is grossly damaged), atrophy of testis and calcification. Retrograde simple orchidectomy is advocated by many surgeons in order to prevent spread of infection. An inguino scrotal incision is preferred and the cord is to be ligated after opening the inguinal canal. The testis with its covering is enucleated from the scrotum after proper hemostasis. A drainage tube should be inserted inside the scrotum before the wound is stitched in layers. Hemostasis by coagulation diathermy is advocated by many surgeons but chances of postoperative wound infection is more due to presence of devitalized tissue in scrotum.

ACUTE MASTITIS

Clinical Features

Acute filarial mastitis is second common filariasis in females next to filariasis of limbs. Normally males do not suffer from filarial mastitis. Acute filarial mastitis occurs after the age of 15 years but it is more common between the age of 25 to 40 years. Lactating mothers suffer more than nulliparous women. Acute filarial mastitis is very rare after the age of 70 years as well as in atrophic breast. However no breast is immune to such an acute manifestation. Normally acute filarial mastitis is a common accompaniment of acute axillary lymphadenitis of same side.

Pain, fever and swelling are the common presentations of acute filarial mastitis. Patients of mastitis complain pain and discomfort in breast and axilla of same side. This pain is constant and dragging in nature being referred to back epigastrium and along the medial side of arm and forearm. This pain is exaggerated by coughing and sneezing as well as movement of breast. The patients get relieved after support of breast like acute orchitis. The intensity of pain increases depending on the severity of the disease. In many cases it is seen this pain is localized to upper and outer quadrant of the affected breast. Constant and throbbing type of pain with insomnia indicate breast abscess in late cases.

Like acute filarial fever the patients may suffer from rigor with fever and vomiting. The fever may continue for 2 to 3 days depending upon the use of antibiotics and severity of infection. Some patients may not present like acute filarial fever except some rise in temperature and pulse rate. Pain and fever almost go hand in hand. As soon as the infection becomes localized due to treatment or due to body immuno responsive process the fever subsides and the breast starts swelling.

There may be edema of breast either localized or generalized. Normally the upper and outer quadrant is more prone to suffer due to more amount of breast tissue present in this quadrant. The nipple, areola and skin of the breast may be edematous and congested. There may be dimpling of skin due to lymphatic edema which mimics the picture of peaud orange of carcinoma breast. The breast may be pendulous. This edema is pitting in character in acute cases. The breast is tender and there may be local rise in temperature. The skin may give a cord like feeling due to lymphangitis and the breast tissue may be edematous and lobulated. The breast tissue may be freely mobile but in late cases some restriction in mobility may be present due to adhesion to pectoralis major muscle. When the infection becomes localize to one sector the mass will be indurated, firm in consistency and tender. The axillary tail of spencer may be enlarged and feel like a separate swelling in the axilla. On squeezing the breast, serous and hemorrhagic fluid may come out through the nipple. In late and untreated cases ulceration of skin and areola and breast abscess are possible. In effective and improper use of antibiotics in breast abscess changes the abscess to a firm mass called as "antibioma". This antibioma confuses with carcinoma breast clinically until it is excluded by excisional biopsy. Repeated attacks of filariasis in breast produce elephantiasis of breast in late cases.

The lymph nodes in axilla may be enlarged, tender and mobile. These are usually discrete but repeated infections help in matting the lymph nodes. Biopsy of the lymph node will reveal the presence of adult worms of filariasis in it.

In acute cases there may be leucocytosis and neutrophilia. There may be eosinophilia in 5 to 15 percent of cases. In late cases lymphocyte count may increase. Night blood for microfilariae may be positive in many cases.

Differential Diagnosis

Fibroadenosis of Breast

The fibroadenosis of breast is an alternation in the physiological process of breast parenchyma at the time of evolution (menarche) or involution (menopause). The pathological changes are like micro-cystic formation, papillomatosis, adenosis, epitheliosis and fibrosis. The patients complain of pain and discomfort without rigor and fever. This pain is increased during each menstrual period. The breast is multi-nodular which are tender and palpable only by pulp of the fingers but not by palmar surface of hand. A part or whole of the breast may be involved without involvements of skin, areola and nipple. There may be greenish fluid discharge through nipple. The axillary lymph nodes may or may not be enlarge and tender.

Mondor's Disease

This is thrombophlebitis of superficial veins of breast as well as anterior chest wall without any definite cause. There may be subcutaneous cord like swellings which are nodular and partly tender. The skin may be adherent to it and feel like lymphatic permeation in case of carcinoma breast. Absence of fever and enlargement of lymph nodes exclude from filariasis of breast.

Carcinoma Breast

An antibioma may confuse with carcinoma breast always unless excluded, after excisional biopsy. The carcinoma breast is a painless process unless involves the chest wall or there is distant metastasis. Retraction of nipple and skin are usually found in carcinoma of breast and such is absent in antibioma. History of irregular and ineffective use of antibiotics after an acute attack of mastitis, is present in antibioma and such is not found in carcinoma breast. The mass may be tender and firm in consistency in antibioma and shape may be regular in periphery of the swelling. However, it is very much difficult to exclude carcinoma of breast from antibioma unless excisional biopsy is done.

Treatment

Antibiotics, antihistamines, vitamins and hematinics are the treatment of choice in acute mastitis. As soon as the acuteness subsides, antifilarial drugs should be advised in order to prevent further attacks and complications (see antifilarial drug chapter). Like acute orchitis use of support relieve the pain in acute mastitis. The patients should be advised to use brassiere regularly which prevents complications like elephantiasis and abscess formation.

Any breast abscess should be drained out as soon as possible and as much as practicable. Simple use of antibiotics without drainage helps in formation of antibioma. Submammary or Langer's incision is choiced during draining the breast abscess. All loculations should be broken up in order to facilitate the drainage. Use of gauge or globes drain is advocated till the abscess cavity closes by granulations.

In case of antibioma the mass should be excised and send for histopathological examination in order to exclude malignancy. Extracapsular excision or lumpectomy is advocated by many surgeons in order to maintain the beauty of the woman. If the mass is big enough and the patient is beyond menopause simple mastectomy may be performed following which the mass is to be subjected to histopathological examination (Frozen section biopsy). In young patients if elephantiasis of breast is observed then mammoplasty is advised. Replacement is preferred over reconstruction mammoplasty. First simple mastectomy is done and followed by replacement mammoplasty for cosmetic purpose.

ACUTE RETROPERITONEAL LYMPHANGITIS

Clinical Features

Acute retroperitoneal lymphangitis is defined as inflammation infection of lymphatics of retroperitoneal space in which pain, loss of appetite, vomiting, distention constipation and absence of bowel sound are common features therein. This disease can affect *per se* or may be an accompaniment of genital fila-riasis or inguinal lymphadenitis. Ascending infection of lymphatics is more common than occurring as such. Males are more sufferers than females. Patients are usually above the age of 40 years and present with acute onset of pain in lower abdomen, fever, constipation and vomiting.

Like acute filarial fever, rigor comes first than fever. Pain in abdomen and fever go side by side. Usually pain begins at lower abdomen more towards iliac fossa. Gradually this pain is referred to lumbar region, back and epigastrium. There may be pain in inguinal region due to involvement of inguinal lymph nodes. This pain is constant and pin pricking in character. In female patients, pain may start from hypogastric region due to salpingo-oophoritis. Some patients complain of spasmodic pain in abdomen due to pelvic peritonitis which leads to subacute obstruction in large gut. Constipation is a common feature in patients of retroperitoneal lymphangitis. In late cases, there may be absolute constipation due to development of paralytic ileus. Due to absolute constipation the patients develop distension of abdomen. This distension is uniformly marked in abdomen and for this reason respiratory distress is a complaint by many patients. In late cases of paralytic ileus, the pain disappears except respiratory distress. In chronic cases there may be diarrhea more of mucus and chyle (chylous diarrhea).

Vomiting with dehydration may be present in many patients as stomach is the loudspeaker of abdomen. The vomiting is mainly due to super-addition of gastritis and pylorospasm. Many pathologists advocate that due to interconnection of lymphatics of pyloric region and that of peritonium the infection is lodged immediately in this zone for which spasm develops in pylorus leading to vomiting. Hence, in infection of any adbominal organ vomiting is a feature. In late cases anuria and uremia are possible. Due to repeated attacks of retro-peritonial lymphadenitis, the tributaries of cisterna chyle become obstructed and thereby chylous ascites and chylous diarrhea are caused. Patients pass more of potassium in mucus and protein.

There may be mild anemia, rise in pulse rate, dehydration and foul smelling breath. The tongue may be coated as in all cases of septicemia and abdominal infection. On palpation of abdomen, there may be tenderness throughout the abdomen. Bowel sound is absent or if present may be like bells at evening pealing. This tone is high pitched note which occurs in every ten to thirty seconds due to overflow of fluid from one distended loop to another. Radiologically the abdomen shows distended loops of intestine with multiple fluid levels.

The hematological picture of this disease is similar to that of acute peritonitis (bacterial) in which polymorphonuclear cytosis along with eosinophilia may be seen. Night blood for microfilariae is positive in most of the cases. Ascending lymphangiography may show blocks in lymphatics.

Differential Diagnosis

Acute Appendicitis

Pain, vomiting and fever are the earliest symptoms in appendicitis. This pain begins at umbilicus or epigastrium, vague or spasmodic in nature and lastly localizes to right iliac fossa when parietal peritonium is involved. In filarial peritonitis, pain begins at iliac fossa spreads gradually upwards and is referred to lumbar region. In appendicitis the temperature never exceeds 99 to 101°F whereas in this conditions the temperature can reach up to 104°F. The iliac or inguinal group of lymph nodes are free in appendicitis but are primarily involved in this condition. Microfilariae will be absent in blood in appendicitis.

Perforated Peptic Ulcer

Sudden onset of agonizing pain in epigastrium of a peptic ulcer patient without fever (may be accompanying with vomiting) indicates perforation of existing gastroduodenal ulcer. This process undergoes three stages like stage of peritonism, stage of reaction, (or stage of illusion) and stage of peritonitis, obliteration of liver dullness, presence of rebound tenderness, silent abdomen distension, absence of bowel sounds and presence of pneumoperitonium confirmed by radiological investigations, help in the diagnosis of perforated peptic ulcer. Absence of rigor with fever and non-involvement of iliac and inguinal lymph nodes differentiate the condition from acute filarial retroperitoneal lymphangitis.

Treatment

Antibiotics, gastrointestinal decompression and maintenance of electrolytes and fluids are the treatment of choice in early stage.

Combination of streptomycin and penicillin is the antibiotic of choice as both antibiotics combinely act almost a broadspectrum antibiotic. Tetracycline may be given in case the patient is sensitive to penicillin or in resistant cases.

In order to prevent dehydration fluid and electrolytes therapy is essential. Normally 5 percent dextrose saline and 5 percent dextrose solution are given which provide caloricity to the patient as well as fluid and electrolytes. Gastrointestinal decompression by Ryle's tube is provided in order to prevent paralytic ileus. As soon as the patient passes flatus oral fluid therapy may be started. Water and soft drinks like fruit juice should be the first diet of choice.

As soon as the acuteness and features of septicemia subside, antifilarial drugs should be given to the patient in order to prevent further attacks. Some physicians like to give 'Placentrex' or 'Sterodine' with a view to provide energy to the reticuloendothelial system for the production of antibodies hematinics and vitamins should be given to all patients.

Bilateral excision of fallopian tubes may be indicated in patients having repeated attacks of salpingo-oophoritis. Hydrotubation (antibiotics and steroids) is performed in patients where tubes cannot be removed for the sake of fertility. During removal of tubes, at least one ovary or a part of it should be preserved in order to prevent earlier development of atherosclerosis. Biopsy of infected lymph nodes may be performed in case the patient is subjected to laparotomy. Drainage may be provided to the peritoneal cavity in case of pyoperitonium.

ACUTE ARTHRITIS, ACUTE SYNOVITIS, ACUTE MYOSITIS AND ACUTE TENDINITIS

Clinical Features

A joint includes bones taking part in formation of joint and soft tissues like capsule, synovial membrane ligaments and muscles with their tendons. As all the above tissues are involved in the formation of joint infection of one invites involvement of other tissues. For this reason the four conditions are described in this chapter.

Commonly the joints of lower extremities like knee and ankle, suffer from filariasis. Accordingly the quadriceps fumoris, Gastrocnemius and solius with tendoachalis tendon are involved in filariasis. Pain and swelling are usual presentations of these conditions.

In arthritis and synovitis, pain is felt in movements of joints and muscles, responsible for such movements. Pain is felt at the beginning of movement and gradually reduces at the joint becomes free. This is only marked at the initial stage of this disease. The pain becomes constant when there is heavy effusion like hydroarthrosis or pyoarthrosis due to stretching of the capsule. The synovial membrane of tendon sheath or bursae when involved may fluctuate due to effusion. Local tenderness is marked very well. Sometimes there may be itching of the part with congestion due to angioneurotic edema. As soon as there is effusion to the joint space the limb takes the functional position in order to provide maximum space in joint cavity and to relax the capsule and synovial membrane. There may be mild fever or the patients may present like acute filarial fever from the beginning. Bony ankylosis and contracture of muscles may be possible due to pyoarthrosis and lymphangitis of muscles respectively in repeated attacks. Fixed deformity is observed in limbs due to recurrent infection of joint and muscles. Wasting of muscles is seen due to disuse of the limbs in long standing cases. The draining lymph nodes may be enlarged and show features of infection like pain, swelling and tenderness. In malnourished patients involvement of bone ends leads to osteomyelitis and osteochondritis. This condition may be an accompaniment of filariasis of limbs.

The hematological and histopathological picture in this condition looks like acute lymphangitis and lymphadenitis. Microfilariae are cultured in the fluid aspirated from the joint cavity and bursae.

Treatment

Antibiotics and Antihistamines

Like all infections antibiotics and antihistamines should be administered systemically. Tetracycline or chloramphenicol are the antibiotics of choice. Hematinics and vitamins should be given in order to support the reticuloendothelial system.

Aspiration

The aspiration of joint is used for therapeutic as well as diagnostic purpose. For therapeutic purpose aspiration of joint reduces the pain and tension of joints thereby limiting the stretching of ligaments and capsule of the joint. For diagnostic use the aspirated fluid should be subjected for culture and sensitivity. All aseptic precautions should be observed in order to prevent spread of infection to a non-infected joint cavity. This is the only disadvantage of aspiration.

Aspiration and Injection

Some surgeons prefer to inject antibiotics like penicillin, streptomycin or tetracycline with or without steroid soon after aspiration by the same needle. Steroid prevents future fibrosis and development of osteoarthritis. Repeated injections of antibiotics should be avoided as systemic use fulfils the purpose equally.

Arthrotomy and Drainage

If there is pus during aspiration and radiologically there is involvement of bones then arthrotomy is the procedure of choice. The joint should be irrigated with sterile normal saline mixed with antibiotics. During closure of joint a drainage tube may be left in extra synovial space for 24 hours. Some surgeons avoid to put a drainage tube in joint space.

Arthrodesis (Ankylosis)

In repeated joint infection which is beyond antibiotic control the infected bone ends may be excised and allowed for fusion. The joint should be immobilized in functional positions as given in Table 5.1.

Table 5.1: Immobilization of joint in accordance with different functional positions.

Joint	*Knee*	*Ankle*	*Hip*	*Elbow*	*Wrist*	*Shoulder*
Position of immobilization	5 to 10° flexion is allowed in order to clear the ground during walking	At right angle to leg	20 to 30° flexion with a mild abduction and rotation	90° extension right and 135° extension in left, in order to reach the natural openings	5 to 10° Dorsiflexed	40 to 50° abduction and 25° external rotation

Antifilarial Treatment

To all cases antifilarial treatment should be given in order to prevent further attacks of filariasis. The patients should be under repeated interval therapy of such drugs.

Chronic Presentations

chapter 6

LYMPHANGIECTASIS (SYNONYM-LYMPH-VARIX)

Definition

Lymphangiectasis is defined as a condition in which the lymphatics become dilated, tortuous and incompetent. An abnormally dilated lymph node is called as lymphadenovarix.

Etiology

The lymphangiectasis occurs either congenital (primary) or acquired (secondary). In congenital type the lymphatics fail to canalize in proper way for which there is distal dilatation. This is either present at birth or develops late in life. The congenital lymphangiectasis may be associated with congenital arteriovenous fistula and with chylous reflux. In acquired type due to repeated infections particularly in filariasis, tuberculosis or fungal infection the lymphatics are obstructed leading to lymphangiectasis. Commonly lymphangiectasis seen in scrotum, inguinal canal, limbs, breast and retroperitoneal space.

Clinical Features

Lymphangiectasis presents as a gradual swelling which is soft in consistency. Like hemangioma or varicose vein the swelling is compressible. The swelling is fluctuant as it contains lymph in dilated space. This swelling shows impulse on coughing when it is connected with abdomen. Like varicocele of cord, it may feel like bag of worms in scrotum. Multiple blebs or vesicles occur in skin when there is infection and block as in the lymphangitis. These blebs contain lymph when ruptured lead to lymphorrhea. This condition is commonly seen in scrotum and in limbs. Patients of lymphangiectasis may present with acute manifestation of filariasis as seen in lymphangitis and lymphadenitis. It is observed that the swelling increases in size during each acute attack. As soon as the acuteness subsides the swelling reduces in size but does not come to normal condition. Chylous reflux or backflow of milky chyle occurs in conditions when there is block in cisterna chyle. Cutaneous fistulae are seen when there is rupture of lymphatics to outside. Commonly chylorrhea occurs in back with lymphedema. Lymphangiectasis occurring in inguinoscrotal region mimics the feature of inguinal hernia and surgeons unable to diagnose it preoperatively. Lymphangiectasis occurring in femoral triangle confuses with saphaneous varix except the color of the skin which is not a definite sign in a colored person. Multiple cord like feelings or bag of worms with uneven swelling occur if breast is involved. The draining lymph nodes are also palpable and features of infection are observed in these lymph nodes. In repeated attacks one of the lymphatic channel dilates and lymph collects in a cystic space. This condition is known as hydrocele of breast. Histologically it resembles like cystic hygroma (Hydrocele of neck). Similarly, if this thing occurs inside the scrotum it is designed as hydrocele of scrotum. Here the tunica vaginalis testis may or may not be free of hydrocele. Encysted hydrocele of cord bears similar pathology although congenital non obliteration of processes vaginalis may play a role. Repeated infection causes abscesses formation and calcification of cystic wall which can be shown by X-ray picture (Fig. 6.1, Plate 2).

Treatment

Excision is the treatment of choice. Whenever it is present over inguinal region and confuses with inguinal hernia the inguinal canal is to be exposed and the lymphatic tissue is to be excised, care being taken to avoid damage to testicular artery and vas. It is essential to excise the tunica vaginalis testis of same side as there is possibility of development of hydrocele due to damage to lymphatics. This manoeuvre should be performed either through the same incision or through a separate incision over scrotum.

Ligation and excision of fistulus tract in chylous reflux is advised where lymphedema does not improve. Antifilarial treatment improves the lymphatic edema in some cases. In cases of lymph varix at femoral triangle a transverse incision over saphaneous opening is to be made and care should be taken to avoid injury to femoral vessels and femoral nerve. Submammary incision or Langer's incision is usually given if lymphatics cyst is to be enucleated from breast. Submammary incision avoids exposure of scar and the incision of choice for cosmetic purpose. The abscess if any should be drained before enucleation is planned in order to prevent further attacks. The use of sclerosing agents is no more in vow.

Preoperative as well as postoperative treatment by antifilarial drugs is mandatory (see antifilarial drug chapter).

CHYLURIA

Etiology

Chyluria is a condition in which patient passes milky urine mixed with blood due to block in thoracic duct or cisterna chyle. The urine contains more of chyle which contains fat globules. Thereby the urine looks like milk. The most common cause of obstruction is either due to filariasis or tuberculosis. In addition to the above conditions chest injury or spinal injury's tumors pressing the duct or cisterna chyle accidental ligation during surgery, mediastinal fibrosis, etc. can cause obstruction of thoracic duct leading to chyluria.

The chyluric urine when kept in a glass for few minutes, settles into three layers. An upper thin layer of fat, middle layer is lymph mixed with urine and deep layer, sediments of epithelial debris, RBC pus cells, microfilariae and other cells. This urine when mixed with ether or any fat solvent, clears of milky color. In order to confirm the diagnosis the patient should be given 100 gm of fat mixed with 1 gm of confectioners green dye (D and C Green No 6) by mouth and the urine is collected after 12 to 24 hours. This urine will be uniformly green and containing fat.

Clinical Features

Commonly the patients are worried with milky color of urine. Sometimes the urine may be whitish red, or whitish yellow due to presence of blood or bilirubin respectively. This urine always stains the area where the patients micturate which is a common complaint. Frequency, urgency and dysuria are also common accompaniments of chyluria due to urinary tract infection. Pain in lower abdomen is equally a complaint of patients of chyluria (strangury). This pain may be continuous or spasmodic in type and may be referred to penis or scrotum. Pain in lumbar region or back indicates involvements of kidneys and ureters. Many patients complain of burning pain over suprapubic region or back after act of micturition. The patients develop hesitancy and at times retention of urine. Clot colic due to long-standing hematuria may be present in many patients. Features of peptic ulcer like vomiting, hyperacidity, loss of appetite and constipation may be complained. Liver may be palpable and tender in some cases. Morning edema of eyelids, edema of face and limbs indicate involvements of kidneys. There may be hypertension.

Hematuria may be microscopic or frank type. There may be terminal or total hematuria. Presence of threat like clots indicates high hematura. Fever is a common complaint in patients. This may follow rigor. Temperature may rise upto 103 to 104°F. Some patients may have evening rise of temperature. Normally there is 2 to 3°F rise in temperature. Pulse rate increases above 90 always. Sweating from forehead is marked. The temperature may touch the baseline but so far the pulse rate is above 80 it indicates presence of infection in urinary tract. Patients pass pus towards end of micturition (Pyuria). *E. coli* is the most common infecting organism. Less commonly *S.*

fecalis, Stap. aureus, albus, B. proteus, P. aeroginosa. Bacillus proteus and *Staphylococcus albus* are urea splitting organisms for which urine is alkaline in nature. In rest of the infections the reaction of urine is acidic. Persistence of infection invites calculus formation in urinary tract. Latent filariasis of abdominal lymphatics invites recurrent cystitis as well as infection of urogenital system.

Cystoscopic examination reveals multiple vesicles over bladder mucose. This mucose may be congested and multiple erosions with bleeding points may be observed. The trabeculations are edematous. There may be discharge of milky urine through ureteric openings. The ureteric openings may be edematous and there may be ulcerations. Chromocystography should be done by injecting indigo-carmine (7 ml of 0.4%) which will indicate the functional activity of kidneys IVP will show the function and pathology of kidneys. The pelvis, calyces and ureters are visualized by IVP and if there is any stone or stricture can be diagnosed by IVP. The cystoscopic examination may be used for diagnostic as well as therapeutic purpose. Calcification of kidneys or calculus in urinary tract may be visualized by plain X-ray (KUB). The urine not only contains lymph, fat, pus cells, bacteria, epithelial cells, phosphates, protein, red blood corpuscles but also microfilariae. Like all other filariasis there may be microfilariae in night blood and eosinophilia is marked in differential count.

Treatment

Like all filarial conditions antibiotics, antihistamines, vitamins, hematinics and heavy intake of fluids are the earliest treatment of choice. Heavy intake of fluids flushes urinary tract. The antifilarial drugs should be started after excluding tubercular pathology. The antifilarial drugs are to be given in regular intervals for a period of three years (see chapter on antifilarial drugs). Salt intake may be restricted in case of kidney involvements. Low fat is advised.

In resistant cases or long-standing cases chemical cystitis should be induced in order to produce fibrosis of submucosal lymphatics, thereby chyluria can be cured. For this purpose, silver nitrate is choiced. The solutions of silver nitrate in different concentrations are used to wash the bladder as well as ureters up to calyces of kidney.

The concentration is increased from 1 in 50,000, 1 in 25,000, 1 in 15,000, 1 in 10,000 and 1 in 5,000 in gradual intervals. Cystoscopy should be performed in each time of use of silver nitrate. The ureters should be catheterized up to pelvis in order to wash the pelvis by silver nitrate solution. This is to be performed under regional or surface anesthesia. General or spinal anesthesia should not be used in order to avoid injury to pelvis of kidneys. The patients should be under antibiotic cover for a prolonged period which prevents bacterial infection of urinary tract. Urinary alkalization or acidification may be done (in different pH of urine) in order to change the internal environment of urinary system thereby the causative organism cannot grow. Mandalamine and ammonium chloride may be used for the purpose of acidification.

CHYLOTHORAX

Etiology

True chylothorax occurs in conditions when a definite site of obstruction can be localized over thoracic duct. This is possible in injury to thoracic duct or it's tributaries either in accidental trauma or surgical manoeuvre. Spinal injury at thoracic region invites chylothorax as the thoracic duct courses over thoracic vertebrae. Tumors of mediastinum like esophageal carcinoma, bronchogenic carcinoma and lymphatic tumors when obstruct the thoracic duct produce chylothorax. In true chylothorax the effusion is milky and rich in fat and chyle. In pseudochylothorax the effusion looks milky but this is not, due to rich in fat but, presence of calcium phosphate, cholesterol, epithelial cells, pus cells as well as bacteria or parasites. In pseudochylothorax the site of obstruction cannot be localized. Usually the obstruction is in multiple points of thoracic duct. Here, the effusion is produced by filtration through lymphatics due to back pressure at multiple points. Chronic diseases like tuberculosis and fungal infections of lungs and mediastinum produce this type of obstruction. An encysted empyema when ruptures, produces an effusion which looks like milk but this is not rich in lymph although fat may be present. This is mostly due to breakdown of cyst wall (Chyliform effusion). In above, two conditions dye test (using confectioner's green dyes or C and D green No 6 with fat 100 gm) is positive whereas such test will be negative in chyliform effusion.

Clinical Features

Usually chylothorax occurs on right pleural cavity because of course of thoracic duct more towards right than to left. The chylothorax may be generalized or localized (encysted type). Sometimes it may be spontaneous or gradual.

Like empyema the symptoms may be masked by primary infection like fever, rigor, vomiting, restlessness, dyspnea and cough. Increase in malaise with pleural pain, high fever up to 104°F possibly with rigor are of suggestive but sometimes fever may be absent. In massive effusion, there will be dyspnea, cough and pain in chest due to shifting of mediastinum. The pain may be referred to back, neck and upper part of abdomen. There may be loss of appetite and constipation. There may be rise in rate of respiration and pulse. The intercostal spaces of affected side are full and do not move with respiration. The fluid may track intercostally and appear as a fluctuant subcutaneous swelling termed as "empyema necessititis". The trachea and apex beat may be deviated to opposite side of effusion. The entire side of effusion will be dull on percussion. The breath sound will be reduced and vocal resonance with vocal fremitus are absent. These may increase above the level of fluid. If a bronchopleural fistula develops the patient may pass large amount of sputum and the chylothorax drains through the fistula. The cough and expectoration are often accompanied by a vile smell to the breath. Reactionary effusion may occur in pericardial cavity. If chyle leaks daily to pleural cavity and if this is removed the patient may rapidly become depleted of protein, fat, electrolytes and fat soluble vitamins. With healing, there is a gross pleural fibrosis with contraction of the hemithorax and scoliosis. This is commonly seen in children. Chest radiography shows complete obliteration of lung shadow as far as there is effusion. Cardiac shadow shifted to opposite side. Mild effusion may be observed in opposite pleural cavity. Aspiration confirms the diagnosis if subjected to microscopic examination.

Microfilariae may be seen under microscope. Fat content may be less in comparison with cholesterol. Dye, if used, can be aspirated if it is a true or pseudo-chylothorax. Hematological picture mimics that of other filariasis.

Treatment

1. General treatment—Like other filariasis antibiotics, antihistamines, hematinics and vitamins given as soon as possible. Ampicillin, amoxillin, tetracycline or gentasporin should be given as the patients show mixed infections. Fluid and electrolytes should be replaced in order to meet dehydration as well as nutrition. Fat soluble vitamins like vitamins A, D, K and E should be given along with vitamin B complex and C in order to replace the loss as well as giving support to reticuloendothelial system respectively. The patient should be restricted of fat intake and loss of protein be replaced orally. Antifilarial treatment should be given as soon as possible.
2. Special treatment (given below).

(a) Aspiration (Thoracocentesis)

Thoracocentesis should be made both for diagnostic as well as therapeutic purpose. The aspiration should be done in a dependent point as possible. Normally 7th to 9th intercostal space in midaxillary or posterior axillary line is selected for aspiration. The aspiration is made in sitting posture under regional anesthesia. Care should be taken to avoid injury to intercostal nerve and vessels thereby preventing hemothorax.

The aspiration is made in selected interval, depending on the amount of collection. Repeated aspiration causes hypoproteinemia and avitami-nosis of fat soluble vitamins particularly A and D. The patient should be always under antibiotic cover.

(b) Pleurodesis

Fusion of parietal pleura with visceral pleural helps in prevention of secretion of chyle. Commonly iodized talc is used for the purpose. This reagent is subjected into pleural cavity through the needle after complete aspiration of chyle. The reagent is usually diluted by normal saline and is kept for half an hour and aspirated completely.

(c) Thoracotomy

In case of not responding to antibiotics and aspiration, thoracotomy with tube drainage is made if there is possibility of empyema thoracic. This procedure is selected at dependent part of chest and care is to be taken to prevent pneumothorax. For this, tube should be fixed to chest wall and air tight water seal mechanism is selected. Patient is tough about respiratory exercise. He may be advised to inflate and deflate a balloon regularly thereby diaphragm moves up and down smoothly. Regular change of bottle with antiseptic solution should be made in order to prevent ascending infection. Bottle connection may be disconnected after assuring complete non-drainage. This can be known from the glass tube provided in the bottle. Gradual shortening of chest tube may be made till the cavity closes completely.

(d) Ligation

Ligation of thoracic duct or its tributaries may be indicated in cases where the above trials fail to achieve the result. Lymphangiography may be done before ligation in order to locate the leak. During thoracotomy dye test can be made to confirm site. In filarial chylothorax, this may not be a routine practice. Pleurectomy is a remote possibility in filarial chylothorax.

ELEPHANTIASIS OF LIMBS

Etiology

Elephantiasis occurs in lower limb more commonly than the upper limb. Portions of limb below knee or elbow are affected by elephantiasis. In some patients, elephantiasis may spread above knee or elbow as far as the trunk. This may be bilateral or unilateral. Sometimes one upper and one lower limb may be affected by elephantiasis either contralateral or ipsilateral side. From teenagers to old are the victims of this disease. This disease is caused by complete block of lymphatics thereby the lymph accumulate in the affected limb at the dependent part. The lymph comes out of lymphatics and enters the interstitial space in subcutaneous region as this space can expand due to elasticity of skin. Contraction of muscles and toughness of deep fascia prevents collection of lymph in deep spaces. "Protein when heated in acidic medium, coagulates". The lymph is rich in protein and the acidic medium is provided by production of lactic acid, pyruvic acid and other acidic metabolites of bacterial infection (Fig. 6.2, Plate 2).

This bacterial infection raises the body temperature for which the proteins in lymph coagulates in subcutaneous space which is termed as blubbery tissue of elephantiasis.

The lymphedema may be present from birth (lymphedema congenita) or at puberty (lymphedema praecox) or in adult life (lymphedema tarda). The congenital noncanalization of lymphatic system produces lymphedema and such a familial condition is found in Milroy's disease. The lymphatic obstruction occurs in filariasis, tuberculosis or fungal infection of lymph nodes. Acute infection of inguinal group can occur in persons walking in barefoot. Trauma as well as surgical removal of lymphatic system (in radical excision) produce lymphedema permanently. Malignant infiltration of lymph nodes produce a fatal lymphedema. (Here mainly filarial cause has been dealt with).

Clinical Features

A patient developing elephantiasis of limb either upper or lower usually suffers from repeated attack of lymphadenitis and lymphangitis of the same limb. Usually it takes a long time to produce elephantiasis of limb (Grade III or Grade IV Pani's edema). In each attack of lymphangitis and lymphadenitis the swelling increases in the limb. Each such attack makes the obstruction worse until the limb becomes grotesquely swollen, the skin folded and wrinkled and coarsened like that of an elephant (hence elephantiasis). There may be brown area of desquamated keratinization. The skin looks like pith of an orange. The edema may be completely or partially non-pitting. The upper part of the swelling may be pitting but the lower part is usually non-pitting. Superficial ulceration, cellulitis and abscess formation may be possible in such a limb. Gangrene partly or completely may be possible in such blubbery tissue leaving the deep tissue exposed. Over granulations or infective granuloma either single or multiple are seen over the limb. In each attack of lymphangitis, there may be lymphorrhea from this limb. Hemorrhage can occur from ulcer areas such a bleeding requires intervention to stop it, as the base of the ulcer is grossly fibrotic. The fibrosis prevents retraction of blood vessels in elephantiatic limb. Although the limb is edematous the movements in joints remain as such in all directions. Rest of the feature akins that of acute filarial fever (Fig. 6.3, Plate 3).

Differential Diagnosis

Elephantiasis Neuromatosa

This condition usually occurs in connection with peripheral nerves particularly with trigeminal nerve (5th cranial nerve). This is a congenital malformation in which histopathological examination shows myxofibromatous degeneration of endoneurium. The skin in this condition is coarse, dry and thickened, resembles that of an elephant. The lymph nodes are normal as well as there is no history of acute filarial fever in this condition. Blood microfilariae will be negative. Biopsy confirms the diagnosis.

Elephantiasis Grecorium

This is a condition seen in lepromatous leprosy. The skin of the face and limbs thickened and nodular. Edema of limbs develops due to anemia and secondary infection. Due to involvement of peripheral nerves like ulnar, radial, lateral popliteal there may be deformity of hand or foot like clawhand, wristdrop, footdrop, etc. There may be lionine facies and atrophy of testes. The breast may be enlarged (Gynecomastia). In nose (depressed nasal bridge, perforation of septum) and eye (lagophthalmos, exposure keratitis, madarosis and iridocyclitis, etc.) deformities are seen in such condition. Skin smear shows abundant of AFB (*Mycobacterium leprae*).

Elephantiasis Chirurgens

This is a condition seen, following radical mastectomy. Due to removal of lymphatics of axilla the arm becomes edematous and skin is thickened as in elephantiasis. This condition can occur in patients subjected to radial operation for carcinoma breast where the axillary lymph nodes are removed. The swelling appears at a period varying from many months to some years. Like filarial fever, there may be signs and symptoms infection of lymphatics in the limb. Patients subjected to radiotherapy are more prone to develop elephantiasis chirurgens.

Pretibial Myxedema

This is a condition seen in hyperthyroidism where mucin like deposits occur under the skin of pretibial region. The skin is thickened and edema is nonpitting. The skin looks like the pith of an orange. The patients usually have exophthalmos and other eye signs of hyperthyroidism. The hair is coarse and the leg becomes cyanosed when exposed to cold. LATS, BMR and PBI are increased in this condition. The lymph nodes are normal and question of fever with rigor does not arise in this condition.

Other Edemas

There can be edema of limbs in conditions like congestive cardiac failure, constructive pericarditis, anemia and hypoproteinemia, cirrhosis of liver, tuberculosis and malignancy. Here, the edema is usually pitting and responds to diuretics very well. The skin does not akin the pith of an orange. Treatment of the condition relieves the edema. Edema is usually bilateral.

Treatment

The elephantiasis of limbs do not respond to medical treatment alone at all. However, antifilarial treatment by antibiotics, antihistamines, hematinics, vitamins and antifilarial agents prevent the further attacks of acute filarial fever and lymphangitis. Diuretics and use of elastic bandage may be helpful. Many surgical procedures have been tried and still under active trial. No definite method has been as yet proved to be centpercent successful. Since the discovery of causative parasite by Sir Patrick Manson in the year 1877. In China, surgeons are still in the process of investigation to achieve the desire goal. Out of many surgical methods the following are in consideration.

Charle's Operation (Flaying Operation)

The aim of this operation is to remove the blubbery tissue as far as the muscles and to cover the raw area by skin graft from the same limb. "Skin is the best dressing and living tissue is the best antiseptics". An improvement on this method is to bury the skin on the whole length of limb like a Swiss cake role so as to create lymphatics in longitudinal direction. No area should be left without covering by skin graft. Skin graft can be given in two or three sittings in order to avoid chronic ulcer and over granulations. If any ulcer is present then it is like that patient gets repeated attacks of acute infectious of filariasis. The hemostasis can be maintained by using an Esmarch tourniquet and general anesthesia is usually preferred.

Kondoleon's Operation

The aim of this operation is to remove the deep fascia so as to connect the two spaces as a result lymph can flow from superficial space to deep space. Multiple longitudinal strips of deep fascia are removed under general anesthesia through longitudinal incisions. Here the blubbery tissue is left as such. However, the swelling does not subside at the same time prognosis of the condition after this operation is not satisfactory.

Handley's Operation

The aim in this method is to create lymphatics in longitudinal direct between the affected limb and the center of drainage like axilla or inguinal region. Multiple threads are to be kept under the skin of affected limb surrounding which lymphatics develop. The result of this operation is still doubtful.

Gilli's Graft

Here the greater omentum of abdomen is brought with the pedicle attached to its sight and kept either in axillary or inguinal region under the skin with an intention to connect the said lymphatics with that of abdomen. This operation is not satisfactory as well.

However, no operation is as yet satisfactory except excision with grafting as in Charles's operation.

ELEPHANTIASIS OF SCROTUM AND PENIS

Clinical Features

The elephantiasis of genitalia in male is second common elephantiasis next to that of limbs. Adults are common sufferers of this condition. This can be seen in the age of teens but never seen below teens. A patient before developing elephantiasis of scrotum or/and penis must have suffered repeated attacks of inguinal lymphadenitis. Many patients suffer from elephantiasis of limbs along with this condition. Scrotum is first to suffer than the penis. Like lymphangitis and orchitis the patients present with all the features of these conditions. Pain and swelling are the earliest complaints. Like orchitis, pain starts from scrotum and is referred as far as back and lumbar region. This pain is relieved after support of scrotum. The edema starts from the most dependent part of scrotum and gradually spreads upwards as far as penis and inguinal region. This edema can involve the skin of lower abdomen particularly of hypogastrium and as far as anus. The skin is thickened like that of limb elephantiasis. The penis may twist on its own axis and the prepucial apperture becomes edematous. The glans buried inside for which it is difficult to retract the penis. Twisted and edematous penis looks like the horn of a ram (Hence Ram-horn penis). The penis may be buried completely inside the scrotum and there be, excoriation of skin of scrotum due to contact of urine. The inner layer of prepuce is free from edema. The cords may be thickened and there may be hydrocele or chylocele of tunica vaginalis testis. The transillumination test is always negative due to thickening of skin, even if there is clear fluid in tunica vaginalis testis. The TVT may calcify in prolonged case involving the epididymis. In non-treated cases, there may be chance of development of cellulitis, abscess and gangrene of scrotum. Autogangrene is seen in many acute cases where the testes are exposed to outside like the clapper of a bell. In such condition, it is difficult to differentiate if from Fournier's gangrene of scrotum. The inguinal lymph nodes are normally palpable and enlarge in such conditions. The scrotal abscess if treated early does not invite such condition. Pyocele of TVT may be an accompaniment of gangrene of scrotum. Lymphorrhea occurs due to rupture of lymphatic vesicles of scrotal skin. Sometimes there may be lymphatic cyst inside the scrotal tissue known as hydrocele of the scrotum and this when infected called as scrotal abscess (Fig. 6.4, Plate 3).

Differential Diagnosis

Fournier's gangrene—The idiopathic gangrene of scrotum is known as Fournier's gangrene. It is an avascular infective gangrene. First infection is caused by scratching and followed by ischemia of scrotum due to edema and leads to necrosis of skin of scrotum. There may be pyrexia, edema of scrotum, and gangrene. The penis is not usually involved. The testes are exposed to outside when the scrotum becomes completely gangrene. The inguinal lymph nodes may be tender and palpably enlarge.

Treatment

Medical Treatment

Like all filariasis antibiotics, antihistamines, hematinics and vitamins should be given in early stage of filariasis. As soon as the acuteness subsides antifilarial treatment started (See chapter on antifilarial drug). This treatment should be given in an interval of three months for a period of three years in order to prevent the relapse.

Surgical Treatment

Excision of all edematous and blubbery tissue and covering the raw area by skin grafting is the treatment of choice. A longitudinal incision should be given on dorsal surface of penis as far as Buck's fascia. Many surgeons like to start exposing the shaft of penis from prepucial opening. The penis is exposed completely till the root of penis is reached. Care should be taken to avoid injury to dorsal vessels and ligament of penis. Then this incision is extended surrounding the scrotum between healthy and edematous skin. The entire edematous skin of scrotum, blubbery tissue, septum of scrotum, fat and fascia of scrotum, are excised by exposing the urethra outside. Care must be taken to avoid injury to urethra. Many surgeons like to keep a catheter inside urethra, thereby injury to urethra can be avoided. The sacs of testes are to be excised if there is hydrocele or chylocele. Complete hemostasis is made by ligation or by diathermy. The scrotal wound is to be closed by interrupted stitches after putting the testis as well as a drainage tube in the most dependent part. If the testes cannot be accommodated inside the existing scrotal skin then tunnels may be made on the anteromedial part of upper thigh through the scrotum and both testes may be placed in this tunnels on their respective sides. Many surgeons like to excise one testis thereby other testis can easily be kept inside the existing scrotal skin because scrotum is the thermoregulating organ for testes. A testis when kept in the thigh, is prone to injury always. Then the skin near root of penis is to be transfixed to root of penis by interrupted chromic catgut stitches thereby the penis will not retract back. A partial thickness skin graft should be given over penis to cover the raw area of penile wound. Bowesman advocated to cover the penis by using the inner layer of prepuce but the penis becomes edematous like a drumstick as there is no lymphatic connection of prepuce to inguinal lymphatics. Many surgeons like to keep a catheter in bladder for 72 hours but this is useless as this is my personal experience that urination easily occurs although there is postoperative edema of glans penis. Patients should be instructed to avoid contact of urine with the dressings given over wound of penis. Movement should be encouraged after 6 hours of operation. The patients should be kept under antibiotic cover for 10 days after which the dressings are removed by careful soakage with normal saline to avoid the skin grafts to give way.

ELEPHANTIASIS OF VULVA

Clinical Features

This is a very rare condition of filariasis. The females above forty are usual sufferers of this condition. This condition is usually unilateral but may be bilateral. Like other filarial condition repeated acute lymphangitis leads to this condition. The edema involves the skin of labia majora and the adjacent parts but not the labia minora. Like other elephantiasis the skin is thickened and looks like the pith of an orange. The vaginal orifice is closed if bilateral manifestation occur. The inguinal lymph nodes may be enlarged and tender during acute presentations. Like elephantiasis of scrotum, urination is not affected in any form. The clitoris and labia minora remain normal throughout the condition. The rest of the features mimic that of elephantiasis of scrotum.

Treatment

Like elephantiasis of other organs, medical treatment is first advised to the patients. Antibiotics, antihistamines, vitamins and hematinics are to be given to prevent further attacks. Excision of edematous and blubbery tissue along with construction of labia majora after skin grafting is the procedure of choice in this condition. Care should be taken to avoid injury to anal sphincter during excision of edematous skin of perineum. In old patients, excision with primary closure if permitted is advocated to avoid delay.

Silent Presentations

chapter 7

HYDROCELE OF TUNICA VAGINALIS TESTIS

Etiopathology

Hydrocele of tunica vaginalis testis (commonly called as hydrocele) is a condition of collection of transudate inside itself. This condition can occur in any age group starting from birth to death in old age. Hydrocele occurring in females in inguinal canal is known as hydrocele of canal of nuck. Hydrocele is commonly seen in adult age group although no age is immune to such condition. Hydrocele may be unilateral or bilateral. accordingly, hydrocele is classified as (pathologically):

A. Congenital type
B. Acquired type
   1. Primary or idiopathic
   2. Secondary.
      - Acute diseases like orchitis, funiculitis.
      - Chronic diseases like TB, malignancy, filariasis, syphilis, etc.

Anatomically hydrocele may be classified as:

Vaginal Hydrocele

In this type the collection of transudate is within the tunica which is confined to scrotum only. This type of hydrocele is commonly seen (Fig. 7.1, Plate 4).

Infantile Hydrocele

This is a rare type of hydrocele in which the tunica is extended up to deep inguinal ring entering through inguinal canal. Such a hydrocele is not necessarily be present in infants only. The tunica bears no connection with peritoneum.

Congenital Hydrocele

Here, the tunica of hydrocele is continuous with peritoneum and the opening is narrowed at deep inguinal ring. This hydrocele can disappear when the patient lies horizontally. Such a hydrocele, although having connection with peritoneal cavity, does not present with inguinal hernia.

Encysted Hydrocele

This type of hydrocele is a localized collection of fluid in tunica present in relation to cord. This may be present at external ring or inside inguinal canal. Sometimes it may be present on the course of cord inside abdomen. Such a hydrocele is free from testis.

Hydrocele-En-Bisac

This is a rare condition of hydrocele where the tunica resembles that of infantile type but this is biloculated due to constriction at the neck of scrotum. Both the loculi are intercommunicated. At times, there may be multiple septa inside the tunica thereby this becomes multiloculated hydrocele but characteristically all are intercommunicated.

In some cases (5%), there may be inguinal hernia on the side of hydrocele particularly in case of vaginal type. Normally, tunica contains 3 to 5 ml of fluid inside it. This prevents friction in testis during movements. This fluid is a balanced of continuous secretion as well as absorption of tunica vaginalis testis. Hence, fluid can collect in tunica due to:

a. Excessive secretion following infection of testis and its surroundings (Orchitis, funiculitis, epididymitis, traumatic orchitis, etc.), such a hydrocele is known as secondary hydrocele. Tuberculosis of epididymis (30%), malignant tumors of testis (10%), syphilis of testis can present with hydrocele which is commonly lax in type.

b. Lack of absorption may be possible due to damage to the endothelium of tunica vaginalis. The exact cause of damage to endothelium is still obscure, hence known as primary hydrocele.
c. Due to combination of both, a and b.
d. Lymphatic drainage when blocked, leads to hydrocele which counts about 80 percent cause of hydrocele in tropics. The most common cause of lymphatic obstruction is filariasis although surgical trauma accounts only 0.2 percent following repair of inguinal hernia. There may be collection of chyle in this obstruction which is called as chylocele of tunica vaginalis testis (Fig. 7.2, Plate 4).
e. Communication with peritoneal cavity causes hydrocele as in congenital type. The entire peritoneal secretion gravitates into the tunica.

Children suffering from TB peritoneum present with this type of hydrocele commonly. The hydrocele fluid commonly contains water, salts of sodium, potassium and calcium, albumin (6%), cholesterol and fibrinogen. This fibrinogen is characteristic of this fluid, when mixed with blood can coagulate easily. For coagulation, factors are required which are present in blood and such are not seen in hydrocele fluid. Hence, fibrinogen helps in coagulation only when other factors are available nearby. The fluid is amber colored and specific gravity is 1.022 to 1.024. fat, cholesterol, microfilariae, pus cells, RBC and high proteins are seen if there is obstruction to lymphatics by filarial manifestation. This is seen in chylocele. Due to collection of fluid there is stretching and thinning of tunica and skin. Constant pressure over testis may produce atrophy of this organ. Repeated low grade infection of tunica may help in deposition of fibrins over testis and its coverings, thereby the tunica becomes thickened. Calcification may occur in long-standing cases. Compensatory hypertrophy of cremasteric muscles, seen in many cases due to heavy weight of the organ. Spontaneous hemorrhage may occur into this fluid causing hematocele which clots within very short period. Old clotted hematocele is usually spontaneous in origin although minor or major injury can produce the similar result. Repeated infection of testis may change the hydrocele to pyocele unless treated properly.

Histopathological examination of tunica shows damage of endothelium, undue fibrosis and infiltration of chronic inflammatory cells like plasma cells, lymphocytes and histiocytes. Testicular fibrosis with infiltration of chronic inflammatory cells are also seen in long-standing cases. These features are seen more in peripheral zone of testis than in center. In idiopathic cases, only thinning of tunica and mild fibrosis are observed without infiltration of chronic inflammatory cells. The skin of scrotum looses its elasticity and there is hypertrophy of dartos muscles. Though this muscle is hypertrophic but functionally it is too weak to recoil back to its previous condition. Hence, skin excision should be mandatory into all cases of sizeable hydrocele thereby looseness of skin can be corrected.

Clinical Features

Transillumination test positive and to get above the swelling are the hallmarks of hydrocele. Almost all hydroceles are translucent. Absence of such character indicates any of the pathology like thickened tunica, hematocele, pyocele, chylocele or thickened skin. The swelling is usually scrotal type unless it is hydrocele-en-bisac or congenital type. One can easily get above the swelling by palpating cord and nothing but the cord. Normally the swelling is globular or pyriform in shape and soft in consistency. The swelling may be firm and tense due to heavy fluid inside. Sometimes there may be herniation of tunica, through dartos like a separate cyst. The swelling is free from skin unless infected. Normally testis is placed posterior to the swelling which is marked for its sensation. Fluctuation is demonstrated in all cases unless old clots are present (old clotted hematocele) which confuses with malignant tumors. The penis may be placed centrally in bilateral condition or may be deviated to one side in unilateral condition. Sometimes the penis may be burried inside the scrotum like in elephantiasis. The cord and vas may be thickened and beaded at places due to repeated lymphangitis. Pain may be complained of, in occasions of infection, or else hydrocele is a painless condition. For this reason patients do not mind for such swellings in scrotum even to the end of life. In congenital hydrocele the swelling may disappear slowly when the fluid enters the peritoneal cavity but sudden rise in pressure or blocking of opening by a patch of omentum at internal ring may not allow the fluid to run into peritoneal cavity. This hydrocele gives impulse on coughing due to its connection with peritoneal cavity and for which it confuses with inguinal hernia. But unlike inguinal hernia transillumination test is always positive in congenital hydrocele. To get above the swelling is not possible in this hydrocele. The swelling in encysted type is always separated from testis but attached to cord. Hence, it moves along with movements of cord. If the swelling is confined to inguinal canal, manual pressure or rise in intra-abdominal pressure during coughing or sneezing dislodges the swelling from its native place and recoils back to its position when the pressure is over. Such a swelling confuses with inguinal hernia except the swelling is fluctuant and translucent.

Complications

Rupture

Minor injury over a tense hydrocele (or at times spontaneous) can rupture the tunica which requires immediate intervention. Sometimes the hydrocele is cured automatically due to absorption of fluid via dartos after perforation. Surgical intervention helps in preventing hematocele formation.

Hematocele

The hematocele may be traumatic or spontaneous. Sudden onset of pain and increasing in swelling of a hydrocele following injury indicates hematocele when the swelling is not translucent. Sometimes the hematocele may be old and clotted, one which may be difficult to differentiate from malignancy of testis. Testis becomes atrophic in old hematocele due to pressure. Recent hematocele should be treated as an emergency condition in order to save testis. Orchidectomy is indicated in old hematocele and where the testis is atrophic. During orchidectomy, condition of other testis and age of the patient along with presence of children should be taken into consideration (Fig. 7.3, Plate 4).

Pyocele

Repeated infection of testis and its tunica can change the transudate to exudate. Pain, tenderness, hectic rise in temperature, enlarge and tender inguinal lymph nodes, congestion and redness of scrotum indicate pyocele formation. The skin of the scrotum may be adherent to tunica at places and may be indurated. Early needle aspiration prevents pyocele formation and can save the testis from excision. Aspiration of tunica reduces the tension from blood vessels thereby circulation of the part increases, as a result early repair and cure are possible. The disadvantage of aspiration is traumatic hematocele formation and infection may spread from skin to inside. This can be prevented by observing asepsis. On balance the advantages outweigh this theoretical disadvantage.

Calcification

Repeated low grade infections of testis and tunica cause thickening of the coverings of testis by fibrosis. Over fibrotic tunica, calcium phosphate is deposited to calcify the tunica which can be casted radiologically. Calcification of testis, epididymis and vas causes obstructive azoospermia and infertility in males.

Treatment

Surgical treatment is a treatment of choice. Cirrhosis of liver, nephrotic syndrome, bleeding disorders like thrombocytopenic purpura, hemophilia and nontreated diabetes mellitus are conditions in which surgery is contraindicated. In diabetes mellitus patients of hydrocele can be operated after the blood sugar is controlled after insulin therapy and such treatment should continue till the wound heals completely.

Excision of Skin

Excision of redundant skin of scrotum is mandatory to all cases of hydrocele irrespective of unilateral or bilateral. The skin should be excised in such a way that both testes should be accommodated in the artificial scrotum, without leaving any space at all. By excising the skin, the testes do not hang downwards for which post operative pain is much less. Secondly, excision of skin gives an opportunity to know the pathology of both sides. Thirdly, when the normal testis is being exposed one can avail the opportunity of doing a minimum like eversion of tunica so that the patients may not face trouble for the same disease anymore. It is also seen that patients, whose skin is not excised during hydrocele operation are more prone to develop elephantiasis of scrotum. The incision should begin at least 1 to 1.5 cm below the root of penis as result no injury will be produced to penis. Care must be taken to avoid injury to urethra during excision of septum.

Lord's Operation

This operation is indicated in hydrocele cases where the amount of fluid is less than 5 ml. The aim of this operation is to reduce the area of secretion and at the same time traumatization will be much less. No space is left behind the testis for collection of blood. The tunica should be opened just opposite to testis and multiple gathering stitches are to be given in such a way, the tunica will gather on the circumference of testis like a bicycle rim. Plain catgut (1/0 or 2/0) should be used for the purpose.

Jaboulay's Operation

The aim of this operation is to expose the area of secretion to that of absorption. The amount of secretion continue as before in this operation but dartos being a muscle, absorbs all the secretion of exposed tunica. The tunica is incised well away from the testis and fixed behind the testis by one or two interrupted stitches. The cord should not be tightened too much in order to strangulate the testis. Complete hemostasis should be observed before closing the skin. A drain should be given in order to avoid hematoma formation. Continuous stitches of tunical margin is no more in practice nowadays.

Excision of Tunica

Complete excision of tunica from the margin of testis removes the source of secretion of hydrocele fluid. Sometimes a rim of tunica can be left near the margin of testis for eversion so that the posterior surface of testis can be covered by tunica. Complete hemostasis should be made before closing the tunica and drainage tube should be placed inside the scrotum at least 48 hours to avoid hematoma formation.

Problems During Operation

1. During opening the sac, care must be taken to avoid injury to testis. Here confirmation is to be made by palpating the testis which is firm and solid. Tunica looks glistening at the same time soft and cystic in consistency.
2. Regarding hemostasis, plain catgut is commonly used for the said purpose, but coagulation diathermy can be used. The danger of diathermy is to invite infection as it leaves many devitalized tissues inside scrotum. Continuous stitches round the margin of tunica is more in practice nowadays. Interrupted stitches should be given for hemostasis of tunical margin.
3. Sometimes the tunica involves the cord as high as possible. During dissecting the tunica from cord the inner layer is to be separated

from outer layer of tunica thereby injury to cord vessels can be avoided. Blunt dissection by scissors is always advisable.

4. Sometimes the tunica is so much thickened, it becomes a problem for eversion. In such cases excision of tunica is the method of choice. Hemostasis may be done by diathermy only.
5. Multisaculated tunica should be excised as far as possible. After excision, eversion should be made to avoid recurrency of hydrocele because one obliterated sacule may enlarge to behave like a hydrocele.
6. Sometimes pyocele is discovered during operation and in such condition opposite testis should not be opened to avoid spread of infection. Some surgeons advocate the opposite testis can be operated under sensitive antibiotic cover. The pus should be sent immediately for culture and sensitivity. Orchidectomy should be made of the pyocele side before operating the hydrocele side.
7. Chylocele and hematocele should be treated in similar line, except in testicular atrophy orchidectomy should be performed.

Postoperative Complications

Hemorrhage

The hemorrhage may be primary, reactionary and secondary. Primary hemorrhage is seen in cases when operated under local anesthesia. For primary hemorrhage the wound should be opened immediately and the bleeding points to be ligated under direct vision. Reactionary hemorrhage is seen following general or spinal anesthesia. As soon as the blood pressure rises there is heavy oozing from the wound. This hemorrhage occurs within 48 hours of operation. Prior to correction of hypertension and bleeding disorders, use of drainage tube, tight bandaging (for 12 hours) and use of styptics can prevent this problem. Secondary hemorrhage is caused by infection of wound. This is mainly due to hematoma formation due to lack of drainage. The penis becomes edematous if there is hematoma inside the scrotum. Use of antibiotics, observing complete asepsis and use of drainage tube prevent such complication.

Retention of Urine

Nearly 2 to 3 percent of patients face this complication. Heavy intake of fluid, avoiding use of morphine, and loose bandaging can prevent this complication. Early ambulation, suprapubic hot and cold compress and heavy intake of fluids can overcome this condition. Failure of conservative treatment invites catheterization to correct the disorder. Spasm of sphincter urethrae is the cause of acute retention of urine.

Wound Infection

Hematoma formation and lack of asepsis invites wound infection in post-operative cases. Patients, of diabetes, pyocele, chylocele and orchitis who were not treated sufficiently before, are likely to suffer from this complication. The internal end of drainage tube should be sent for culture and sensitivity to know the exact bacteria and to which antibiotic they are sensitive. Preventive antibiotics can be used to all cases. Combination of penicillin and streptomycin will always have some advantage unless patient is sensitive to it. The abscess, if formed, should be drained as soon as possible. Stitch abscess does not require drainage. Local hot compress helps in early healing. The wound at the drain sight should last to heal. Discharge of transudate occurs after hot compress through stitch wounds and drain area which does not require any treatment except consolation to the patient.

Secondary Infertility

Azoospermia seen after hydrocele operation due to accidental ligation of vas or involvement of vas in heavy fibrosis and calcification. This is a rare complication. Sometimes infertility is a coexistence with this condition which is detected after post-operative marriage.

To all post-operative cases antifilarial drugs should be given in full course, in order to prevent post-operative attacks, of filarial orchitis and elephantiasis of scrotum. (see chapter on antifilarial drugs).

TROPICAL EOSINOPHILIA

Synonyms

Tropical pulmonary eosinophilia, eosinophilic lungs, tropical eosinophilic asthma, Weingarten's syndrome.

Definition

It is an allergic condition caused by filarial worm characterized by persistent eosinophilia and pulmonary signs and symptoms of infection such as cough, expectoration, rhonchi, crepitation, etc.

Etiology

The most common cause of tropical eosinophilia is filariasis. The filarial worms when produce allergic manifestations, the hemopoietic system responds by producing excess of eosinophilis. Thereby, there is infiltration of eosinophilis, into lung parenchyma. Other agents like drugs, parasitic infections of GI system (ascariasis, ankylostomiasis), skin diseases (Pemptigus, Psoriasis, etc.), Polyarteritis nodosa, malignant diseases like Hodgkin's disease can produce the similar condition in lungs. Recently, it is studied that tubercular allergenes are also responsible for this condition.

Clinical Features

The patients may present with indefinite symptoms of cough and chest pain particularly in ribs. Occasionally, accidental diagnosis occurs due to investigations for some other disease. There may be some irregular history of asthmatic attacks and sometimes episodes of urticaria or angioneurotic edema can occur. The asthmatic attacks occur at night and are usual presentation. This asthma comes in paroxysm. The patients complain of frontal headache, persistent chest pain which is constricting in type. There may be tenderness over ribs. Paroxysmal sweating occurs after each attack of asthma. Examination of chest reveals rhonchi and coarse crepitation, more marked on the basal parts of lungs. The apical zones are free from any sign of infection. Radiologically, the lungs are clear but occasionally hilar congestion with prominency in bronchovascular markings are observed. Rarely there may be discrete rounded mottling marks seen in lung field more in basal zone. Sometimes this may confuse with miliary tuberculosis in which sputum is AFB positive. Sputum when subjected for microscopic examination shows excess of eosinophils without AFB. Hematological picture shows rise in eosinophils (more than 30 to 80%) and total count is more than 15,000 (Leukocytosis). Premature eosinophils cells are seen in peripheral blood as well as in bone marrow.

Treatment

Like all other filariasis antibiotics, antihistamines, hematinics and vitamins should be given. As soon as the acuteness subsides, diethyl carbamazine should be given in a dose 6 mg/kg weight for a period of 5 days and similar course should be given after an interval of 4 weeks. Corticosteroid (Prednisolone-Steroid) may help in refractory cases. Aminophylline and adrenaline may be required during asthmatic episodes. Long acting antihistamines should be prescribed in persistent angioneurotic edema.

Other Filariasis

Other filarial infection like loiasis, onchocerciasis, *A. perstans*, *A. streptocerca* and *M. ozzardi* infections are not of great importance. The reader may refer any textbook for these infections.

Antifilarial Drugs

chapter 8

This chapter will commonly deal with the drugs which are in use nowadays against filariasis. The old drugs such as florocid and arseno typhoid are no more in use for which these drugs are not described in this chapter. The specific drugs which are commonly effective against filariasis are diethylcarbamazine and a herbal product asperzine. In addition to specific drugs other adjuvants are also used in filariasis which are given the therapeutic part of this chapter. Asperzine is a herbal product manufactured by the "Phyto-Pharma" of Odisha in the district of Cuttack. This particular medicine is still under clinical trial. In a study of 200 patients treated by this medicine in filarial clinic, at ESI Cottage Hospital, Choudwar, Cuttack, it is observed that this medicine is equally effective against filariasis. The detail of this medicine is described in its chapter. The ESI Corporation of India and Labor Department of Orissa Government were kind enough to help in purchasing this medicine worth Rs. 12,000 in order to establish the truth of asper-zine. (However work was not completed due to my transfer from that hospital because of political involvement of the superintendent of this hospital with whom, I was not pooling well).

DIETHYLCARBAMAZINE

History

During second world war nearly ten to fifteen thousand soldiers were sufferers of filariasis in America. This had created a problem amongst the physicians to cure the condition by suitable drug. The most promising group of drug is the derivative of piperazine which had changed the course of medical treatment of filariasis.

Chemistry

Diethylcarbamazine is chemically NN diethyl, 4, methyl, -1- piperazine, carboxamide.

This drug is commonly available in the salt form of dicitrate which is colorless, crystalline solid with unpleasant taste. This is highly soluble in water Figure 8.1.

Pharmacological Action

The exact mechanism of action of diethylcarbamazine is still obscure but it is thought that this drug sensitises the adult worms as well as microfilariae to the phagocytic action of reticuloendothelial system. Hence, unless the reticuloendothelial system is strong enough to digest the sensitized filarial worms, the drug bears no benefit at all. The diethyl carbamazine causes rapid disappearance of microfilariae of *W. bancrofti*, *B. malayi* and *Loa loa* from blood of human being within 48 to 72 hours of administration. Onchocerca volvulus and other parasites of filariasis disappear from skin and connective tissue but not from nodules. Harned and his associates in 1948 studied the actions of diethylcarbamazine following intravenous administration that this drug increases the blood pressure followed by fall in this pressure. The pressure response is accompanied by tachycardia and peripheral vasoconstriction. In toxic doses, there may be vomiting,

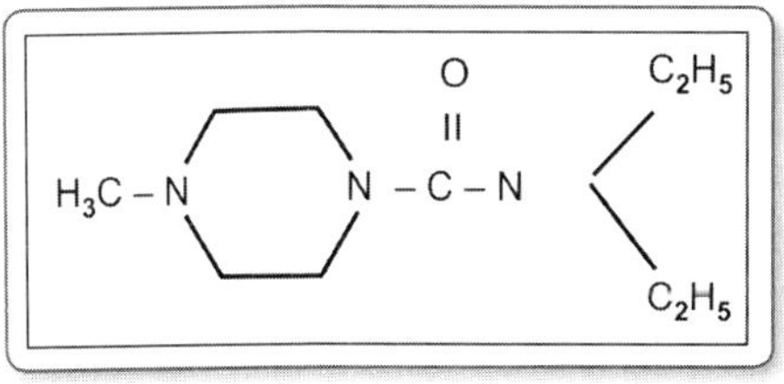

Fig. 8.1: Formula of diethylcarbamazine

muscle tremors and convulsion. As this drug is highly water soluble it can easily get absorbed through gastrointestinal route. After a single oral dose a peak blood concentration appears in 3 hours and this falls to zero within 18 hours. The excretion is almost entirely through urinary system in the form of its metabolites. The compound is distributed almost equally throughout all compartments of human body except in fat. There is little tendency for accumulation when repeated doses are given.

Toxicity

Diethylcarbamazine produces toxicity which is transient but not permanent. The toxicity is mainly headache, general malaise, weakness, pain in joints, anorexia, vomiting and nausea. Some patients complain of neuritis and diarrhea. All these features disappear when the drug is withdrawn. Intravenous or intramuscular administration may cause reeling of headache, vomiting, heaviness in occipital region blurring of vision, hypotension and general weakness. The loss of appetite remains for a prolonged period. Sometimes Jarisch-Herxheimer reaction occurs after use of diethylcarbamazine. This may be due to sudden liberation of endotoxins by adult worms of filariasis following phagocytic action by reticuloendothelial system. This reaction includes edema of skin, increase in previous swelling, angioneurotic edema of lips, skin and anal region, increase in tenderness of lymph nodes, popular rash and hyperpyrexia up to 102° to 103° F. There may be leukocytosis and eosinophilia in this reaction. This reaction is transient which responds to antihistamines. The eosinophilia that occurs in filariasis is intensified following diethylcarbamazine therapy in early days but subsides towards late days of the treatment.

Indications and Contraindications

The indications of diethylcarbamazine are:

1. Filariasis by *W. bancrofti* and *B. malayi*
2. Loiasis

3. Onchocerciasis
4. Infections by *A. streptocerca, A. perstans* and *M. ozzardi*
5. In tropical pulmonary eosinophilia
6. In liver fluke infection
7. In toxocariasis.

This drug may be given in malaria along with chloroquine whose action is potentiated after addition. This drug has no specific contraindication only when the patient cannot tolerate. In such cases this drug may be started with a small dose initially and the dose is increased gradually. In order to prevent reactions antihistamines should be added in each dose of the drug. For this reason, many preparations are marked with a combination of antihistamines in this drug.

Preparation and Therapeutic Use

The diethylcarbamazine citrate is commonly marked as banocide or hetrazan. This is available in form of tablets, liquid and injections. The tablets may be 50 to 100 mg. The product is stable even under conditions of high temperature and humidity. Sometimes combination preparations are available along with antihistamines and steroids. Tablets and injections are marked in this preparation. In order to prevent gastric irritations and as an adjuvant therapy to peptic ulcer patient, antacids are combined with this drug. In tropical pulmonary eosinophilic patients, mucolytics and smooth muscle relaxants are combined with this drug which is beneficial to patients. Use of steroid should be judged carefully and diabetes should be excluded before use of such combination.

Use in Filariasis

Normally, 2 mg/kg weight to a maximum of 300 mg per day in three divided doses are given after each meal. This drug should not be given in empty stomach. Some physicians advise to start one dose on first day, two doses on second day and calculated three doses from third day onwards with a total course of three weeks. Such a treatment is advised only to exclude the sensitivity of patients to this drug and to prevent allergic reactions. But this treatment has no extra benefits as allergic reactions are observed in mid part of treatment. Some surgeons advise to repeat the treatment in usual dose at an interval of 3 months for a period of 3 years. Hence, it is said 3 doses a day for 3 weeks and to repeat 3 monthly for 3 years ("Rule of 3"). For mass treatment with the objective of reducing microfilaremia to subinfective levels for mosquitoes the dose is 2 mg/kg weight three times daily after meals for 7 days. As per World Health Organization report of 1967, a space dose of 6 mg/kg weight should be given once a week or once a month which gives as good an effect as daily dose. This is less likely to cause adverse reaction. Antihistamines should be given till the drug is in use. Hematinics and vitamins should be added during the course of treatment in order to give support to reticuloendothelial system. Cortiocosteroids (Prednisolone) can be used in refractory and late cases which prevents fibrosis and development of elephantiasis.

In loiasis, the dose is 4 mg/kg weight three times daily for a period of 10 days. If repeated courses are required to produce cure, there should be a gap by a period of 3 to 4 weeks. In onchocerciasis this drug is given in a dose of 0.5 mg/kg weight as in a schedule of filariasis and can be increased up to 1 to 2 mg/kg weight for a period of 21 days. Local use of corticosteroid ointment should be started in the involvement of conjunctive. In the initial treatment, systemic reaction may be provoked by massive destruction of microfilariae and adult worms. In such cases, dose should be lowered or the drug may be stopped temporarily. Relief of these symptoms is afforded by the use of antihistamines but exceptionally corticosteroids may be required. Once the initial reactions have subsided, continued treatment does not provoke further reaction at all.

ASPERZINE

History

This product is manufactured by "Phyto-Pharma" a pharmaceutical limited of Orissa in the district of Cuttack. This is herbal product. Primarily this was practiced by the tribal populations of Koraput and Sambalpur in the state of Orissa. The people used to the crude nature of this preparation.

Chemical Composition

Each 5 ml, contains liquid extract of:

Streblus Asper	1: 1–1.0 ml
Argyreia Speciosa	1:1.0–0.5 ml
Liquorice IP–0.2 ml	
Symplocos 1:1–0.1 ml	
Chloroform Spirit	IP–0.07 ml
Alcohol content	× 3% V/V
Flavored syrup base	qs
Total solid 45 to 50% W/V	

Each capsule contains Chlorpheniramine maleate in addition to the contents of liquid except alcohol and syrup.

Pharmacological Properties

The exact pharmacodynamics property of asperzine is still obscure. Both microfilariae and macrofilariae disappear from body after 6 weeks of treatment. Microfilariae disappear from peripheral circulation after 72 hours of treatment but can appear again on discontinuation of the treatment. This preparation bears an irritation property to stomach and other parts of gastrointestinal system. It manifests the latent peptic ulcer for which sufficient precautions should be taken before use of this medicine in peptic ulcer patients. In heavy dose of this liquid preparation produces rise in blood pressure, insomnia and sweating from limbs.

Sometimes Jarisch-Herxheimer reaction like reactions are observed during treatment with asperzine. There may be increase in edema, itching, fever, sweating from limbs. This reaction is transient and disappears after use of antihistamines. Sweating from affected limb is an indication of response to the treatment for which it is a good sign. Eosinophilia tends to normal after 7 days use of asperzine.

Toxicity

The toxicity is marked in 5 to 10 percent cases of treatment by Asperzine. The most common toxicity of Asperzine is anorexia, pain in epigastrium, hyperacidity, nausea, vomiting and constipation. Some patients complain of diarrhea following use of this medicine. Reeling headache, insomnia, heaviness in chest and epigastrium are seen in some patients. Features of polyneuritis and sweating from limbs are observed in 2 percent of cases under treatment. Capsule is less toxic than liquid.

Preparations and Therapeutics

Liquid and capsule preparations are marketed by the farm. 100, 200, and 450 ml phial of liquid preparations are available. 10 ml of such liquid is to be given three times daily after meals for a period of 6 weeks. One capsule can be given in one dose three times daily for a period of 6 weeks. The medicine can be repeated in a period of 15 days interval. For tropical eosinophilia the course is 7 days.

(However, more chemicoclinical study is required to establish the properties of asperzine and it's value in the treatment of filariasis). Some physicians are using L-tetramisole as preventive major M filariasis. It is said that L-tetramisole produces immunity against filariasis. Chloroquine potentiates the action of antifilarial drugs if added during treatment.

BENZOPYRONES

Pharmacology

The benzopyrones are a large group of substance which have many pharmacological property in the human body. Out of 25 numbers tested so far one known Coumarin in proved to be best in reducing high protein edema.

Chemistry

The structure of Benzopyrone is shown in Figure 8.2.

Pharmacodynamics

The pharmacodynamics response of Coumarin is its ability to reduce the capillary fragility and increasing the permeability in lymphatic channels. Coumarin provides alternative pathway in the lymphatic system for the removal of excessive plasma proteins from the tissue by activating the macrophages. In addition the macrophages present in a chronic high protein edema are often inactive and filled with lipid.

Coumarin reactivates this lipid Coumarin has no noticeable effects on the plasma protein level in the blood. This is because the number of macrophages at the site of high protein edema are greatly increased even up to 150 times more than normal as is their proteolysis. Their proteolysis far outweigh that of the macrophages else where in the body. Coumarin has no anticoagulant property.

Pharmacological property: Coumarin is a white amorphous fat soluble substance having sulty taste and absorved within four hours

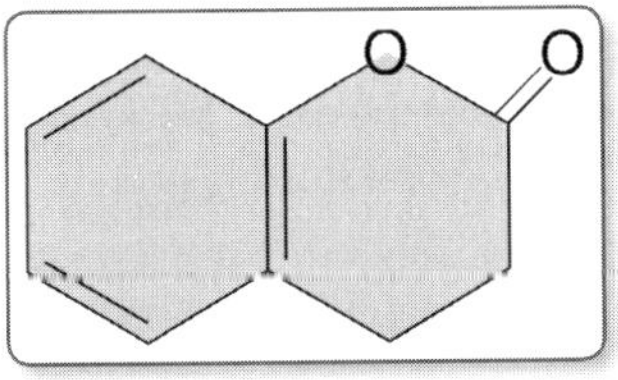

Fig. 8.2: Coumarin (5,6 benzo-α-Pyrone)

in stomach and intestine. The action of Coumarin can be detected about four hours after administration and maximal at 24 hours. By reducing edema it prevents secondary infections of bacteria and fungus. Oral absorption Coumarin is high. Over 80% is found in the urine within 24 hours and 90% of Coumarin is excreted as metabolites. Coumarin mainly metabolized by liver in form of glucoronidation. Its distributed in all organs like brain, heart, lungs, liver, spleen and all connective tissue.

Indication of Coumarin

The main indications of Coumarin is lymphatic edema primary as well as secondary of filarial origin. It can be used as an adjuvant in traumatic and surgical edemas. Hemorrhoidal bleeding can also be controlled by Coumarin.

Doses

About 0.8 mgs/kg weight orally subjected to a maximum dose of 400-mgs per day. Coumarin can be used intravenously with a dose of 0.25 mgs/kg weight. Local application in form of ointment and powder is possible.
Side effect of Coumarin: Side effect of Coumarin are limited about 0.5% of patients who may experience nausea, vomiting, diarrhea or constipation anorexia, dizziness and occasional headache. The side effects are temporary and may required additional medical supports for its remission.

Contraindications

There is no specific contraindication for a use of coumarin. Patients of acute gastric ulcers can take the drugs along with specific treatment. This drugs should be a voided in early pregnancy and in edema in toxemia of pregnancy.

Precaution

Use of Coumarin in children below 12 years is to be made in supervision of a qualified medical person experience in such treatment.

Other drugs like Benzopyrones hydroxyethyl rutine are best known for their use in venous disease but they also reduce many form of high protein edema including lymphedemas Figure 8.3.

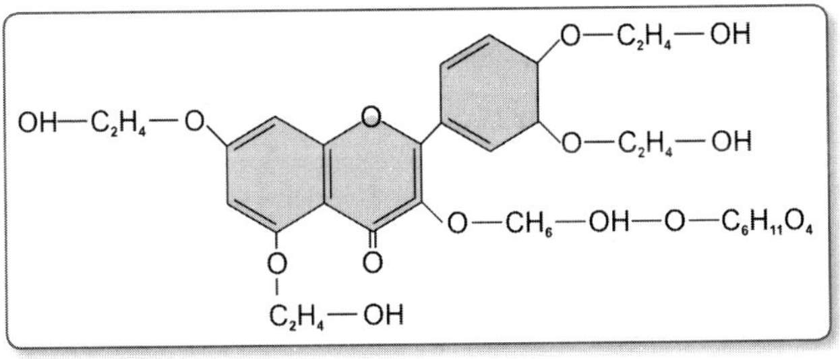

Fig. 8.3: Benzopyrones hydroxyethyl rutin

chapter 9

Complex Physical Therapy

There are many physical therapies advocated now-a days in treatment of edema such as manual lymphatic drainage (MLD) use of local ice compress heating with microwaves, compression with mercury and complex physical therapy. However out of all above therapies complex physical therapy (CPT) proves to be the best so far. The CPT is commonly practised by physiotherapists but a general surgeon can do the work as prescribed in the treatment. A course of CPT normally lasts 2 to 6 days in a week. It has four steps of events.

1. Skin care of the edematus area in order to prevent secondary infection and further complications.
2. Special form of massage which assists the lymphatics to help unaffected regions to drain the affected areas.
3. Use of Low—Stretch compression bandage or paddings during the course of treatment in order to imprevent further edema of the affected part.
4. Special exercise to supplement the massage.

SKIN CARE

The treating surgeon should keep in mind that there should not be further infection in the skin of the affected part. The limb should be kept clean and dry. It there is lymphorrhea from the affected limb use of Gentian Violet (1%) once a day, use of local application of Coumarin and closed dressing are of beneficial nature. Uses of systemic sensitive antibiotics are recommended.

MASSAGE

Special lymphatic massage first empties the lymphy of the normal tissue surrounding the edematous region. Then the affected limb is subjected to special massage in the direction of lymph flow. It starts on the part of the limb adjacent to the trunk and gradually more of the limb involved. This type of massage helps in opening of collateral lymphatics of the affected limb. The massage ultimately softens the affected limb.

USE OF COMPRESSION BANDAGE

Use of low stretchable compression bandage on the affected limb during resting hours particularly at night, and working hours helps the reduction in size of edema compression bandage are an essential part of CPT. If used by themselves the lymphedema may stop from becoming worse.

SPECIAL EXERCISE

The patients should be advised to under go physiotherapy of the affected limb by providing training in exercise of the muscles involved in edema. Active exercised is advised during using the compression bandage. If compression garment are combined with special exercise the limb will usually reduced in size. Maintenances of reduction depends upon the patient wearing a compression bandage practicing skin care looking after their limb, treating any infection promptly and preserving with their exercise.

Index